THE ESSENTIALS OF STRENGTH TRAINING FOR SENIORS

A SIMPLE GUIDE TO INCREASE STRENGTH, BALANCE, AND MOBILITY TO PROMOTE LONGEVITY AND IMPROVE INDEPENDENCE

RUSH HEMPHILL PT, DPT, CSCS

CONTENTS

A TOKEN OF APPR

As a small token of my appreciation, I've included
this book and strength training.

**5 Essential Daily Exercises for Posture: Movin
Better Health and Independence**

Good posture is vital for balance, strength, brea
age, maintaining an upright, healthy posture
impossible. These five exercises are desi
muscles, enhance balance, and promote lor
towards better posture, strength, and, ultima

**Click here or scan the QR code to get yo
Exercises for Posture" now!**

Incorporating these five exercises into your
posture, balance, and overall quality of li
tice these exercises regularly to reap the
postural, mobility, strengthening, and ba
strategy to improve your independence
Here's to your health and vitality!

Click here to d

CONTENTS

A TOKEN OF APPRECIATION

As a small token of my appreciation, I've included a free gift to help you succeed with this book and strength training.

5 Essential Daily Exercises for Posture: Moving and Strengthening Your Way to Better Health and Independence

Good posture is vital for balance, strength, breathing, and overall well-being. As we age, maintaining an upright, healthy posture can become challenging, but it's not impossible. These five exercises are designed to strengthen your postural muscles, enhance balance, and promote longevity. Let's embark on this journey towards better posture, strength, and, ultimately, a more fulfilling life.

Click here or scan the QR code to get your free copy of "5 Essential Daily Exercises for Posture" now!

Incorporating these five exercises into your daily routine can help improve your posture, balance, and overall quality of life. Remember, consistency is key. Practice these exercises regularly to reap the maximum benefits. A combination of postural, mobility, strengthening, and balance training can be the most effective strategy to improve your independence and strength and live your best life. Here's to your health and vitality!

Click here to download it now!

INTRODUCTION

In the golden years of life, there is an element of health that often goes unnoticed - the power of strength training. While the benefits of strength training are widely recognized for younger individuals, it is also essential for seniors to participate in such activities. Strength training holds the key to unlocking a realm of potential in terms of health, longevity, and vitality that many seniors may feel is beyond reach.

Strength training, often misunderstood as a pursuit only for the young and athletic, is, in fact, an activity with far-reaching benefits for individuals of all ages, particularly seniors. The benefits of strength training are manifold, from improving bone density to combating the onset of age-related conditions. It is a powerful antidote to the physical frailty often associated with aging and a formidable ally in our quest for longevity and health. It's not just about the body, either. Regular strength training can also work wonders for mental health, helping to keep memory sharp and mood elevated. It aids in increasing muscular strength, enhancing balance, promoting bone health, and improving overall physical function. The purpose of this book is to underline these benefits and more, dispelling any misconceptions you may have.

However, let's be clear: this is not just a book about strength training. It is a guide, a companion on your journey toward improved health and vigor in your senior years. It's a journey of becoming stronger, more agile, and, most importantly, leading a fulfilling and independent life.

As we progress through the pages of this book, we will discuss the principles of strength training, simplified workout routines, safety guidelines, and tips for maintaining motivation together. You'll find practical exercises, everyday scenarios, and specific recommendations that can easily be incorporated into your daily routine.

This book is a testament to the belief that age is not a barrier to strength and that strength training can be a powerful tool for seniors seeking to live their best lives. So, let's get started on this journey together, knowing that every step taken is a step towards better health and a longer, more active life.

1

STRENGTH TRAINING DEMYSTIFIED

Do you remember those effortlessly light movements you made in your youth? The ease of bending down to pick up a fallen object, or the joy of playing with grandchildren without feeling the strain the next day? As we age, these movements can become more challenging, and you may find yourself feeling anxious about the idea of strength training. However, it's more manageable than you might think.

DEBUNKING STRENGTH TRAINING MYTHS

Let's start by addressing the elephant in the room: the myths surrounding strength training for seniors. These misconceptions often deter older adults from taking that first step towards a healthier, stronger life. Let's go through each one and shed light on the reality.

Myth: Strength Training Causes Joint Pain

One of the most common misconceptions is that strength training leads to joint pain. Research actually indicates that regular, controlled strength training can help reduce joint pain and stiffness. One study published in the Journal of Rheumatology revealed that resistance training improved muscle strength, physical function, and disease activity in older adults with arthritis.

Strength training done right can increase muscle strength and flexibility, taking some of the pressure off your joints and reducing the likelihood of pain. It's like oiling a creaky door hinge - the lubrication allows for smoother, less painful movement. Motion is lotion.

Myth: Seniors Can't Build Muscle

Another myth that often circulates is that seniors can't build muscle. This stems from a biological process called sarcopenia, which refers to the loss of muscle mass and strength that can occur with age. While it's true that we lose muscle as we age, it's not true that we can't build it back.

In fact, studies have shown that seniors can still gain muscle mass with regular strength training. A study from the Journal of the American Medical Association demonstrated that even nursing home residents in their 90s were able to increase their muscle strength through light strength training. So, there is always time to start.

Myth: Strength Training is Dangerous for Seniors

The third myth revolves around safety. Many seniors believe that strength training is inherently dangerous and may lead to injuries. However, strength training is safe and can help prevent injuries when done with the proper form and technique.

Strength training can help seniors improve balance and coordination, reducing the risk of falls, which are a leading cause of injury. Moreover, it can improve bone density, reducing the risk of fractures. It's like building a protective fortress around your body, fortifying it against the threats of falls and fractures.

Myth: I'm Too Old to Strength Train

Finally, the most pervasive myth of all: "I'm too old to strength train." This is not a statement of fact but a reflection of a mindset that sees age as a barrier. The truth is that age is not a barrier to strength training. In fact, it's quite the opposite. Whatever your starting point, there are endless possibilities for modifying and performing various strength training exercises to meet your individual needs and abilities.

Research also shows that strength training can have numerous health benefits for seniors, including reducing the symptoms of chronic diseases like arthritis, diabetes, osteoporosis, obesity, and back pain. It's never too late to reap the benefits of strength training. Think of it like starting a new hobby. Just as you can learn to paint or play an instrument at any age, you can start strength training at any age, too.

Throughout this book, we'll explore these concepts in more depth, providing you with the knowledge and confidence to embark on your strength training journey. With each myth debunked, I hope you feel more empowered and ready to take the next step toward a healthier, stronger you.

Remember, the goal isn't to become an Olympic weightlifter or body-builder. It's to improve your quality of life, to make everyday tasks easier, and to enjoy your golden years to the fullest. So, let's put these myths to rest and move forward with open minds and determined hearts.

STRENGTH TRAINING VS. OTHER FORMS OF EXERCISE

Strength training holds a unique position in health and physical fitness, but how does it compare to other forms of exercise, such as aerobics and yoga? Each exercise type brings its own set of benefits, and understanding these can help you create a well-rounded fitness routine.

Aerobics and Cardiovascular Health

Aerobic exercises, also known as cardio, works your heart and lungs, improving your cardiovascular health. Activities like brisk walking, cycling, swimming, or dancing fall into this category. Cardiovascular exercises strengthen the heart, increase lung capacity, aid in weight management, and elevate mood by releasing endorphins, the body's natural mood boosters.

However, while aerobics help your cardiovascular system and can aid in weight loss, they do not specifically target the loss of muscle mass that occurs as we age. That's where strength training comes in and provides benefits.

Yoga and Flexibility

Yoga, a practice originating from ancient India, is another form of exercise popular among seniors. It combines physical postures, breathing techniques, and meditation to enhance flexibility, balance, strength, and mental well-being. Yoga can be an excellent exercise choice for improving joint mobility and promoting relaxation.

While yoga can help build some strength and stability, it might not provide the level of resistance needed to increase muscle mass and bone density significantly. Strength training fills this gap, especially in muscles or movements not performed in yoga.

STRENGTH TRAINING AND MUSCLE HEALTH

Strength training involves working your muscles against some form of resistance, be it your body weight, dumbbells, resistance bands, or even household items like water bottles. As your muscles work to overcome this resistance, they adapt and grow stronger.

Unlike cardio, which primarily benefits the heart and lungs, strength training targets multiple components of fitness. It improves muscular strength, power, and endurance. Additionally, unlike many other forms of exercise, strength training helps stave off sarcopenia, the age-related loss of muscle mass, keeping you strong and independent as you age.

Furthermore, strength training has a unique benefit called "after-burn" or Excess Post-exercise Oxygen Consumption (EPOC). This means that even after you've finished your workout, your body continues to burn calories, supporting weight management. In the long term, this leads to improved metabolism, making it easier to keep off excess body fat and maintain lean muscle.

Strength training, aerobic exercises, and yoga each offer unique benefits. Cardiovascular exercises improve heart health, yoga enhances flexibility and promotes relaxation, and strength training builds muscle and bone strength. Incorporating all three components into your fitness regimen will provide a holistic approach to health and well-being.

Let us remember that the focus of this book is strength training, not because other exercises aren't beneficial, but because strength training is often overlooked and misunderstood, particularly among seniors. It's time to shine a spotlight on this crucial component of physical fitness.

Throughout this book, we'll explore strength training in-depth, providing you with the knowledge and tools you need to integrate it into your life. We'll cover everything from the basics of strength training to creating a personalized workout routine, with a particular emphasis on safety and injury prevention.

So, let's move forward, armed with the knowledge that strength training is safe for seniors and a powerful tool for enhancing health and longevity. With each page, you'll gain a deeper understanding of strength training and its myriad benefits, empowering you to take control of your health and live your best life.

IMPACT OF STRENGTH TRAINING ON AGING BODIES

When we discuss strength training, it's important to remember that its impact extends beyond just muscle health. It also significantly influences other aspects of our physical well-being, including bone density, metabolism, and posture.

Improved Bone Density

Bones are dynamic structures that constantly remodel themselves in response to physical demands. When you engage in strength training, the resistance applied to your muscles translates into stress on your bones, which respond by becoming denser and stronger. This process, known as bone remodeling, can help counteract age-related bone loss, or osteoporosis, that many seniors face.

Osteoporosis can be a significant health concern for many seniors. It is a condition characterized by weakened bones and an increased risk of fractures. It often goes undetected until a fracture occurs, as it is a silent condition that doesn't exhibit symptoms in its early stages. After menopause, the rapid decrease in estrogen levels significantly affects bone density, putting postmenopausal women at a higher risk. However, men are not immune; they can also experience a gradual loss of bone density as they age.

Risk factors for osteoporosis include genetics, age, a history of fractures, certain medications, and lifestyle factors such as smoking, excessive alcohol consumption, and a sedentary lifestyle. A diet low in calcium and vitamin D also contributes to the risk, as these nutrients are crucial for bone health.

To help prevent and improve osteoporosis, a combination of strength training and proper nutrition is vital. Strength training not only increases muscle mass but also puts stress on the bones, stimulating bone growth and improving density. This kind of exercise is crucial for seniors, as it helps maintain the structural integrity of their bones, akin to how a skyscraper needs a solid framework to withstand the forces of nature. Just as the skyscraper's framework is reinforced over time, your bones become denser and stronger with regular strength training, helping to prevent fractures and breaks.

Nutrition plays a complementary role in bone health. A diet rich in calcium and vitamin D is essential for bone formation and maintenance. Calcium is a primary building block for bones, while vitamin D helps the body absorb calcium. Foods high in calcium include dairy products, green leafy vegetables, and fortified foods. Vitamin D can be obtained from exposure to sunlight, fatty fish, and fortified foods as well. Supplements may be recommended for those who cannot meet their needs through diet alone.

The fight against osteoporosis in seniors is twofold: engaging in regular strength training to enhance bone density and following a balanced diet rich in essential nutrients for bone health. By addressing both these aspects, seniors can significantly reduce their risk of osteoporosis and maintain stronger, healthier bones as they age.

Enhanced Metabolism

Strength training also plays a pivotal role in enhancing metabolism. As we age, our metabolic rate naturally slows down, which can lead to weight gain and related health issues. However, regular strength training can help counter this trend.

Muscle tissue is metabolically active, meaning it burns calories even at rest. Increasing your muscle mass through strength training raises your resting metabolic rate, which results in more calories burned throughout the day. It's like having a car with a more efficient engine. Even when the car is parked, it burns fuel more efficiently, just as your body burns calories more efficiently with more muscle mass.

Strength training not only stimulates muscle growth but also boosts fat metabolism by increasing the production of various hormones. This hormonal response further aids in maintaining a healthy body weight and promoting overall metabolic health.

Better Posture and Balance

The benefits of strength training aren't just confined to the internal workings of your body. They also manifest in visible, tangible ways, such as improved posture and balance. As strength training targets various muscle groups, it helps correct muscular imbalances that may contribute to poor posture. In addition, stronger muscles provide more stability around joints, offering increased support, function, and movement.

Consider your body as a ship. For the ship to maintain its balance and navigate smoothly, all parts must work together harmoniously. Similarly, a well-rounded strength training routine ensures all your muscle groups are strong and function harmoniously, leading to improved posture and balance. This not only enhances your physical appearance but can reduce the risk of falls, a common concern for many seniors.

Strength training also improves proprioception, the body's ability to perceive its position in space. This improved sense of body awareness is crucial for maintaining balance and coordination, making everyday activities safer and more comfortable.

The impact of strength training on an aging body is multifaceted, benefitting not just your muscles but also your bones, metabolism, and posture. Regular strength training can help you maintain a healthy body weight, prevent bone loss, improve your physical appearance, and enhance your overall quality of life. Let's set aside any hesitations we may have about strength training. With each weight lifted and each resistance band pulled, we're not just building muscle. We're improving our bone health, boosting our metabolism, enhancing our posture, and ultimately taking control of our health and well-being.

SETS, REPS, AND TERMINOLOGY SIMPLIFIED

Understanding the basic terminology is crucial to fully benefit from strength training. This section will help you understand the meaning of repetitions, sets, and the concept of load and volume in strength training.

Understanding Repetitions

In strength training, a repetition (rep) is the number of times you perform a specific exercise without resting. For instance, if you lift a dumbbell, the action of lifting it up and bringing it down counts as one repetition.

Think about the process of baking a batch of cookies. A single repetition would be equivalent to baking one cookie. The act of mixing the ingredients, rolling the dough, and baking it in the oven represents one complete cycle - one repetition.

In strength training, the number of repetitions performed depends on individual fitness level and goals. As a senior starting strength training, you could start with around 10-15 reps per exercise and then gradually increase either reps or weight as your strength and endurance improve. For example, focusing on correct form and posture during an exercise while aiming for 10-plus repetitions can help you gain proficiency in the movement. As you gain confidence and strength, lower reps and higher weights can be performed if desired.

Deciphering Sets

A set, on the other hand, is a group of consecutive repetitions. Once you've completed the desired number of repetitions, you have completed one set. Using the cookie-baking analogy, baking a dozen cookies would be equivalent to completing one set.

Determining the number of sets you should do depends on various factors, including your fitness level, the type of exercise, and your specific strength training goals. However, a good starting point for seniors new to strength training could be two to three sets of each exercise.

Grasping Load and Volume

Load and volume are two fundamental components of a strength training program. The load refers to the amount of weight you're lifting or the resistance you're working against. If we continue with the cookie-baking analogy, the load would be equivalent to the size/weight of the cookies you're baking. Larger cookies require more dough, just as lifting heavier weights requires more effort.

Volume, meanwhile, refers to the total amount of work you do in your strength training session. It's typically calculated as the number of sets multiplied by the number of reps multiplied by the load. So, if you did two sets of 10 reps with a 5-pound weight, your total volume would be 100 pounds (2 sets x 10 reps x 5 pounds = 100 pounds). In our cookie-baking scenario, the volume would be the total number of cookies you bake, taking into account both the number of batches (sets) and the size of the cookies (load).

In the long term, your goal should be to increase total volume. This should be done slowly and thoughtfully over time. Doing so ensures you are adequately challenging yourself to adapt, leading to strength and muscle gains. Even just adding one more rep in a workout or increasing the load by one pound on an exercise adds up over time.

Understanding these terms can help you structure your strength training workouts more effectively, ensuring you are progressively challenging your muscles without overdoing it. Your goal should be to increase the volume per workout over time gradually. This stress will lead to increased muscle mass and strength adaptations.

With this new understanding of the essential strength training terminology, you are now better equipped to plan and perform your workouts. Remember, the goal is not to lift the heaviest weights or do the most repetitions right from the start. Instead, it's to gradually and consistently challenge your muscles, allowing them to grow stronger over time. Just as baking perfect cookies requires time, practice, and patience, so does building your strength and endurance through strength training.

Now that we've grasped the basic concepts and terminology of strength training, we can confidently move forward. Strength training is a potent technique that can considerably improve your overall health and well-being. It's not an activity reserved for the young or the ultra-fit - it's a practice that anyone, including you, can incorporate into daily life, regardless of age or fitness level. So, let's move forward, step by step, rep by rep, set by set, towards a stronger, healthier you.

2

POWER OF STRENGTH TRAINING FOR SENIORS

P icture the scene: you're walking along a beach, feeling the sand between your toes, and hearing the waves crashing against the shore. You're not concerned about losing your footing or running out of breath. You're simply enjoying the moment, feeling confident and capable. This scene is not a distant dream but a tangible reality that strength training can bring to life. As we delve deeper into the world of strength training, we'll discover how it can boost your independence and longevity, giving you the freedom to live your life to the fullest.

BOOSTING INDEPENDENCE AND LONGEVITY

Increased Mobility

Think about your daily activities. Making a cup of tea, picking up a grandchild, or even getting in and out of a chair. They all require some degree of mobility. Our mobility can decline as we age, making these everyday tasks more difficult. However, strength training can help reverse this trend.

Strength training works by challenging your muscles with resistance, causing them to adapt and grow stronger. This increased muscle strength can significantly improve mobility, making daily tasks easier. It's like having a good pair of walking shoes. With them, you can walk longer and more comfortably, just as with improved mobility, you can move more freely and easily.

Enhanced Daily Functioning

Strength training not only boosts mobility but can also enhance overall daily functioning. It improves muscle strength and endurance, making everyday tasks easier and requiring less effort. Imagine you're carrying a basket of laundry. Increased muscle strength makes this task less strenuous, saving you energy for other activities. It's like upgrading from a manual to a power-assisted steering in a car - the driving process becomes smoother and requires less effort.

Longer, Healthier Life

The benefits of strength training extend beyond improved mobility and daily functioning; it can also contribute to a longer, healthier life. Regular strength training can help manage chronic conditions such as heart disease, diabetes, and arthritis, reducing the risk of premature death. Consider strength training as your personal health insurance. Just as insurance protects against unforeseen circumstances, strength training safeguards your health, helping you to enjoy a longer, healthier life.

In addition, strength training has been linked to improved mental health, better sleep quality, and increased cognitive function. These factors can significantly boost your quality of life, adding not just years to your life but life to your years.

Let's put this into perspective. Imagine you're a gardener tending to a tree. Regular watering and proper care (strength training) will help the tree (you) grow strong and live long. Neglect the tree, and it may not reach its full potential or enjoy a long life. Similarly, regular strength training can help you enjoy a long, vibrant life ripe with potential.

In a similar scenario, imagine there is a drought, and the tree has not received water in weeks. A strong tree (one with a good foundation of strength training, muscle mass, and strength) will more likely be able to withstand the drought and recover faster than a weaker tree (one that does not have optimal strength, bone density, and muscle mass).

So, as we continue to explore the world of strength training, remember the beach scene we pictured at the beginning. Each strength training session brings you one step closer to that reality, empowering you to walk with confidence, enjoy life's simple pleasures, and live your golden years on your own terms.

IMPROVING BALANCE AND REDUCING FALL RISK

Balance-Boosting Exercises

Strength training offers a remarkable advantage in terms of boosting balance and stability, critical components in leading a self-reliant life. Just like a ballet dancer needs exceptional balance to perform, we need balance for almost every movement we make. It's the invisible thread that weaves through each action, from walking to bending to simply standing upright.

Incorporating balance-boosting exercises into strength training can help improve stability, making you steadier on your feet. Imagine exercises like standing hip abductions, which work your lateral hip muscles while challenging your balance. Or, consider a heel-to-toe walk, a simple yet effective exercise that enhances both balance and coordination. These exercises can be important players in a well-rounded strength training routine, helping you maintain steadiness and ward off falls.

Fall Prevention Techniques

Every 11 seconds, an older adult is treated in the emergency room for a fall, and every 19 minutes, an older adult dies from a fall, according to the National Council on Aging. These staggering numbers underscore the importance of fall prevention techniques in a strength training program.

Strength training builds muscle power and enhances proprioception, your body's sense of position. This is crucial for preventing falls. When you lift a weight, you're working your muscles and improving your body's awareness of its movement and position. It's like a GPS for your body, helping you navigate your environment safely and confidently.

In addition, strength training can improve your reaction times. If you stumble, faster reaction times can help you recover quickly and avoid a fall. If you trip but have a faster reaction time and adequate leg strength, you have a better chance of catching yourself to prevent falling than someone with a slower reaction time or weaker leg strength. Think of it as a built-in safety net, ready to catch you if you falter.

Improved Coordination

While strength training is often associated with muscular strength and endurance, it's less known for its impact on coordination. Yet, the ability to coordinate movements is critical for performing day-to-day tasks, from getting dressed to preparing meals.

Strength training necessitates a level of mind-muscle connection, which can enhance coordination. When performing an exercise, your brain and muscles must cooperate to execute the movement correctly. This constant communication between the brain and muscles can improve overall coordination, making everyday activities smoother and more efficient.

Imagine you're playing a piano. Your hands must work in harmony to produce a melodious tune. Similarly, improved coordination from strength training allows your body to function harmoniously, making daily tasks easier and more enjoyable.

Strength training can be a potent tool for improving balance and reducing the risk of falls. By incorporating balance-boosting exercises, adhering to fall prevention techniques, and enhancing coordination, you can navigate your world with increased confidence and grace, making the most of your golden years. So, let's continue to explore the myriad benefits of strength training, one step, one rep, one set at a time.

ENHANCING ENERGY AND VITALITY

Energy-Boosting Workouts

Picture a crackling fire. Its warmth envelopes you, lending an inviting glow to the room. Now, imagine this fire residing within you, fueled by the energy-boosting workouts in your strength training routine. Strength training exercises can keep your internal fire burning brightly, infusing you with energy and enthusiasm to face the day.

Now, let's look at a little basic physiology. A key player in this energy boost is a molecule called adenosine triphosphate, or ATP. During strength training, your muscles break down ATP to release the energy needed for contraction. This process stimulates the body to produce more ATP, which translates into increased energy levels and energy reserves.

Take the leg press exercise, for instance. As you push against the resistance, your leg muscles are hard at work, breaking down ATP to fuel the effort. Subsequently, your body compensates by ramping up ATP production, thus providing you with a reservoir of energy that can last long after your workout.

Improved Stamina

Along with boosting energy, strength training can also improve stamina. Stamina, also known as endurance, is the ability to sustain physical effort over a prolonged period. It's the steadfast horse that carries you through a long journey, the enduring flame that burns steadily.

Strength training builds stamina by enhancing muscular endurance and cardiovascular health. When you lift weights, your muscles learn to tolerate exertion for longer periods. In addition, your heart and lungs work harder to supply oxygen to the working muscles, improving your cardiovascular endurance.

Consider a simple overhead shoulder press exercise. Each time you press the weight up and down, your shoulder muscles contract and relax. Regularly performing this exercise teaches your shoulders and other upper extremity muscles to endure prolonged periods of work, gradually increasing your stamina.

Another scenario is a simple sit-to-stand movement. If someone has low stamina, they may only be able to perform a few repetitions of standing up and sitting down before resting. Conversely, someone who can perform 20 repetitions with ease will have enough energy and stamina to recover quickly and then go on to their next daily activity.

Enhanced Mood and Mental Health

Strength training can do wonders for your mood and mental health. As you lift weights, your body releases endorphins, often called "feel-good" hormones. These endorphins interact with the receptors in your brain to reduce the perception of pain and trigger positive feelings. This benefit can improve mood, sleep, and confidence and decrease overall pain levels.

Furthermore, strength training can enhance self-esteem and self-efficacy. As you watch your strength increase and your physique improve, you'll likely feel a sense of accomplishment and a boost in confidence. It's like learning a new skill. As your proficiency improves, so does your confidence in your abilities.

In essence, strength training can be an effective strategy for enhancing energy and vitality. The energy-boosting workouts ignite your internal fire, while the improved stamina ensures the flame endures. And the enhanced mood and mental health? They add a sparkle to the flame, making it burn brighter.

STRENGTHENING MENTAL HEALTH

Stress Reduction Techniques

In our dynamic world, stress is an all too common experience. From fretting over health concerns to navigating the challenges of aging, stress can take a toll on our mental well-being. However, strength training can act as a potent stress-buster, helping to alleviate the pressures that can cloud our minds.

Engaging in strength training triggers the release of endorphins, which act as natural painkillers and mood enhancers. These endorphins can create a sense of calm and well-being, helping to alleviate stress. Think of these endorphins as your personal stress relief team coming to your aid after each strength training session.

Additionally, the very act of focusing on the movements and techniques involved in strength training can divert your attention from stress-inducing thoughts. It's akin to the concentration required in knitting or painting, where focusing on the task at hand provides a form of mental respite.

Exercise and Improved Sleep

A good night's sleep is like a deep cleanse for your brain, purging it of the day's stresses and preparing it for the next. Many seniors experience sleep issues, including trouble falling asleep and frequent waking up during the night. Strength training can help improve sleep quality, ensuring you wake up feeling refreshed and rejuvenated.

Regular strength training can help regulate your body's internal clock, or circadian rhythm, promoting a healthier sleep-wake cycle. Just as the sun rises and sets at specific times, your body has its own internal schedule, and strength training can help keep this schedule in tune.

Moreover, the physical exertion involved in strength training can make you feel more tired by the end of the day, promoting a deeper and more restful sleep. Think of it as earning your good night's sleep, with each rep and each set contributing to a night of restful slumber.

Boosting Cognitive Function

Our brains are extraordinary organs capable of incredible feats. However, our cognitive abilities can decline as we age, affecting aspects such as memory and attention. The good news is that strength training can help boost cognitive function, keeping your brain sharp and agile.

Strength training is not just a physical endeavor but also a mental one. Engaging in this form of exercise requires concentration, coordination, and planning, stimulating various parts of the brain. Completing a movement is like solving a puzzle, where muscles work together as pieces to form the picture.

One of the key benefits of strength training, particularly in the context of cognitive health, is its role in promoting the release of various hormones and proteins that support brain health. A critical player among these is Brain-Derived Neurotrophic Factor (BDNF), a protein that has a significant impact on the brain's functionality.

BDNF is a member of the neurotrophin family of growth factors, which are essential for the growth, development, and maintenance of neurons. It acts as a fertilizer for the brain, encouraging the growth of new neurons and the survival of existing ones. BDNF is crucial for neuroplasticity, which is the brain's ability to form new neural connections throughout life. This plasticity is crucial for learning and memory, and it helps the brain adapt to new situations or to recover from injuries.

Exercise, including strength training, has been shown to significantly increase the production of BDNF in the brain. During physical activity, the elevated heart rate and blood flow increase the expression of BDNF, particularly in the hippocampus, a region critical for learning and memory. This increase in BDNF can lead to improved cognitive function, better memory retention, and a decreased risk of cognitive decline as we age.

BDNF is also known to have an antidepressant effect. It helps in mood regulation and has been found to be lower in individuals suffering from depression and other mood disorders. Regular exercise can, therefore, play a role in improving mental health by boosting BDNF levels.

In essence, BDNF is a powerful component of brain health, acting as both a protector and enhancer of cognitive function. By engaging in regular strength training, seniors can stimulate the production of BDNF, leading to a multitude of benefits, including enhanced memory, learning capabilities, and overall brain health. Thus, strength training can be considered essential for maintaining physical fitness and cognitive vitality as we age.

Strength training can play a pivotal role in strengthening mental health. It can significantly enhance your mental well-being, from reducing stress to improving sleep and boosting cognitive function. So, let's lift those weights, push against that resistance, and in the process, lift our spirits, push out stress, and pull in a sense of calm and well-being.

That's the end of our exploration in this chapter, but merely the start of your adventure in strength training. As we move forward, remember the power that strength training holds. Harnessing this power can help you lead an independent, vibrant life full of energy and vitality. It can guide you in maintaining balance and stability and act as a beacon, illuminating your path toward improved mental health. So, gear up to lift your life, one rep, one set at a time.

3

BUILDING A SAFE STRENGTH TRAINING ROUTINE

I magine yourself as the conductor of an orchestra. You have the pivotal role of ensuring that each instrument plays its part correctly, harmoniously, and safely. Now, let's apply this image to your strength training routine. As the conductor of your own body, your job is to ensure that each exercise is performed safely and effectively, reducing the risk of injury and reaping the maximum benefits. The key lies in adhering to proper progressive overload and injury prevention principles, focusing on the appropriate form and technique, the importance of warm-ups, and safe exercise modifications.

INJURY PREVENTION PRINCIPLES

Proper Form and Technique

Similar to how an archer must position their body correctly to hit the target accurately, the effectiveness of strength training exercises relies heavily on maintaining proper form and technique. Good form ensures that the right muscle groups are targeted in each exercise, maximizing the benefits of your workout. More importantly, it can reduce the risk of injury that can arise from incorrect movements or overexertion.

Consider the classic strength training exercise: the bicep curl. In this exercise, you lift a weight by bending your arm at the elbow, working the bicep muscle. However, if you swing your arm or use your back to hoist the weight, not only are you reducing the effectiveness of the exercise, but you're also potentially risking injury to those body parts.

To ensure proper form, start with lighter weights, use control, and increase gradually as your strength improves. Keep your movements slow and controlled, resisting the temptation to rush. If possible, perform exercises in front of a mirror to check your form, or consider working with a fitness professional initially to learn the correct techniques.

Importance of Warm-Ups

Before a runner embarks on a long race, they don't immediately burst into a full sprint. Instead, they warm up their muscles with light jogging and dynamic stretching. Warming up is equally important in strength training. It increases your heart rate and circulation, preparing your body for physical activity, loosening up joints, and increasing blood flow to the muscles. This process helps to reduce the risk of injuries and improve your performance.

A good warm-up routine could include five to ten minutes of light cardio, such as walking or cycling, followed by dynamic stretching exercises that involve moving parts of your body through a full range of motion. For example, leg swings, arm circles, or marching.

Safe Exercise Modifications

Just as a tailor adjusts a garment to fit the individual wearer, exercises can be modified to fit your own abilities and limitations. Modifications can make exercises safer, more comfortable, and more effective for you, reducing the risk of injury and ensuring that you're working at a level appropriate for your fitness level and ability.

Take the push-up, for example. It is an excellent exercise for strengthening the chest, shoulders, arms, and core. A traditional push-up is performed in a high plank position, which can be challenging for beginners or those with wrist issues. A safer and less demanding modification would be a wall push-up or a knee push-up, where the upper body is lifted off the floor using the knees as a pivot point.

Remember, every exercise has a modification, and there's no shame in using them. The goal is not to perform the most challenging version of an exercise but to perform it in a way that is safe and effective for you. After all, the benefits of strength training come from consistency and gradual progression, not from pushing beyond your limits and risking injury.

WARM-UPS, COOL-DOWNS, AND THEIR IMPORTANCE

Effective Warm-Up Routines

Consider strength training as an exciting performance and warm-up as the rehearsal preceding the main event. During this rehearsal, the actors - your muscles - prepare for action, rehearsing their roles and getting into character. A well-executed warm-up routine is like this preparatory rehearsal, readying your muscles for the upcoming workout.

A dynamic warm-up is ideal before a strength training session. This should be performed after your initial 5-10 minute cardio warm-up. This involves performing movements that raise your body temperature and heart rate, lubricate your joints, light muscular engagement, and trigger your nervous system's response, preparing your body for physical exertion.

A warm-up could consist of light cardiovascular activities such as marching in place or cycling on a stationary bike, dynamic movements such as marching in place or jumping jacks, and dynamic stretches involving movements such as leg swings or arm circles. These activities increase blood flow to your muscles, warming them up and enhancing their flexibility and efficiency.

Cool-Down Techniques

Once the performance - your strength training session - concludes, it's time for the closing act: the cool-down. The cool-down is equivalent to a gentle, gradual curtain call, allowing your body to transition from the high-energy performance to a state of rest.

A cool-down routine typically involves gradually reducing your pace and performing static stretches, where you hold a stretch for 20-30 seconds. This helps lower your heart rate, cool down your body, and stretch out the muscles that you have worked during your training session.

For instance, you could start your cool-down with a slow walk after a strength training session, gradually lowering your heart rate. Follow this with static stretches targeting the muscles you worked out, such as a doorway chest stretch or a hamstring stretch. These stretches help lengthen the muscles back out, reducing muscle tension and aiding recovery.

Impact on Muscle Recovery

Both warm-ups and cool-downs play an instrumental role in muscle recovery, the process where your muscles repair and strengthen themselves after a workout. They are like the bookends that hold together the story of your workout, each playing a crucial role in ensuring the story unfolds smoothly and successfully.

Warm-ups help prevent premature fatigue during your workout, ensuring you have the stamina to complete your training session effectively. They also may reduce the risk of injuries, which could otherwise sideline you from your workout routine and delay your progress.

Cool-downs, on the other hand, may help reduce muscle stiffness and soreness post-workout. By stretching out your worked muscles, you help alleviate any muscle tension built up during the workout, promoting faster recovery. This could help with decreased stiffness and soreness the following day. In addition, you typically benefit more from stretching after a workout when your body temperature is increased rather than stretching randomly during the day when your muscles and joints are not warmed up. These variables help ensure you are ready for your next workout.

Warm-ups and cool-downs are not mere add-ons to your workout routine. They are integral segments that enhance the effectiveness of your workout and promote recovery. So, as you plan your strength training session, remember to include these critical bookends. They will ensure your workout story unfolds smoothly, effectively, and safely, leading to a successful and rewarding strength training experience.

TAILORING EXERCISES TO YOUR ABILITIES

Let's visualize strength training as a symphony of movements, with every exercise presenting a unique rhythm and tempo. The beauty of this symphony lies in its adaptability, allowing you to modify the rhythm and tempo to fit your abilities and preferences. In this section, we will explore how to tailor exercises to your capabilities by assessing your fitness level, modifying exercises, and progressing at your own pace.

Assessing Your Fitness Level

Before setting foot on the dance floor, a dancer gauges the rhythm and pace of the music. Similarly, before diving into strength training, it's vital to evaluate your current fitness level. This evaluation provides a starting point for your strength training program, ensuring that the exercises are neither too easy nor too challenging.

To assess your fitness level, consider both your physical capabilities and your health history. Physical capabilities encompass your current level of strength, flexibility, balance, and endurance.

For instance, how many flights of stairs can you climb without feeling winded? How far can you reach down to pick up something from the floor? How long can you balance on one leg? The answers to these questions can provide insights into your physical capabilities.

Your health history, on the other hand, includes any past or present injuries, chronic conditions, or health-related limitations. Sharing this information with your healthcare provider or a fitness professional can help identify any necessary exercise modifications,

ensuring a safe and effective workout routine. Consult your health-care provider, such as a physical therapist or physician, before engaging in a new exercise program.

Modifying Exercises

Once you've assessed your fitness level, you can begin to tailor exercises to fit your capabilities. Think of these modifications as adjusting the volume of your symphony, ensuring it's neither too soft nor too loud but just right.

Exercise modifications can take various forms, including adjusting the range of motion, changing the resistance, or altering the position.

For example, if a standard push-up is too challenging, you could perform the exercise with your knees on the floor or with your hands against a wall, reducing the amount of body weight you need to lift. If lifting a certain weight causes discomfort, you could switch to a lighter weight or use resistance bands instead.

Remember, strength training for seniors aims not to push your body to its limits but rather to challenge your muscles safely and effectively. Modifying exercises allows you to do just that, ensuring each workout is tailored to your abilities and goals.

Progressing at Your Own Pace

Now that you've assessed your fitness level and learned how to modify exercises, it's time to consider progression. In the symphony of strength training, progression is like gradually increasing the tempo, adding complexity and intensity to the music.

Progressing at your own pace means gradually increasing the intensity of your workout over time. This could involve lifting heavier weights, performing more repetitions, increasing the number of sets, or reducing the rest time between sets.

However, it's crucial to listen to your body and progress at a challenging but manageable pace. If you feel pain, excessive fatigue, or any other discomfort during or after your workout, it may be a sign that you're progressing too quickly.

It's also important to celebrate your progress, no matter how small. Every additional pound lifted and every repetition performed is a testament to your strength and determination. So, take pride in your progress, knowing that with every workout, you're one step closer to a stronger, healthier you. The key is to stay consistent over time. It is more beneficial to exercise two times a week consistently than attempt four to five times a week but only maintain it for a few weeks before falling off track.

Ultimately, tailoring exercises to your abilities allows you to take charge of your strength training routine. You can ensure your workouts are safe, effective, and enjoyable by assessing your fitness level, modifying exercises, and progressing at your own pace. So, let's continue this symphony of strength training, adjusting the rhythm and tempo to our unique abilities and dancing our way toward improved health and vitality.

THE ROLE OF REST AND RECOVERY

Importance of Rest Days

As we dip our toes into the strength training waters, it's crucial to remember that progress isn't solely about the time spent lifting weights or performing exercises. It also hinges on the periods of rest and recovery that follow those workouts.

Think of it like sowing seeds in a garden. After the seeds are planted, they require a period of rest, a chance to absorb nutrients from the soil, soak in the sunlight, and gradually sprout into seedlings. Similarly, after a strength training session, your muscles need time to repair, rebuild and strengthen.

Incorporating rest days into your training routine gives your muscles this necessary recovery time. During these rest periods, the body goes to work repairing muscle tissue, strengthening the connections between nerves and muscles, and replenishing energy stores. This recovery process is vital for muscle growth and development, making rest days an integral part of your strength training routine. Also, remember that it can take longer for our bodies to heal and recover as we age.

Signs You Need More Recovery Time

As the conductor of your body's orchestra, it's essential to listen to the symphony of signals your body sends, especially those indicating the need for more recovery time.

Several signs can point to inadequate recovery, such as persistent muscle soreness lasting more than 48 hours post-workout, decreased performance levels, prolonged fatigue, or an increased resting heart rate. Other signs could include trouble sleeping, changes in mood, or a reduced motivation to exercise.

If you notice any of these signs, it may indicate that your body needs more time to recover. In such cases, consider taking an extra rest day or incorporating lighter activity days into your routine. This could include taking a 30-minute walk or performing a chair yoga session instead of strength training.

Restorative Activities

While rest days mean taking a break from your strength training routine, they don't necessarily mean being completely inactive. Engaging in restorative activities can support recovery, keeping your body lightly active while providing your muscles the rest they need.

Restorative activities can include gentle forms of exercise that promote flexibility and circulation, such as yoga or tai chi. These activities can help loosen tight muscles and boost blood flow, aiding recovery. Going outside on a walk is an excellent form of active recovery that should be included in a daily routine as well.

Other restorative activities could include:

- Getting a massage to relieve muscle tension.
- Practicing deep breathing exercises to promote relaxation.
- Taking a warm bath to soothe sore muscles.

Remember, rest and recovery are not sidelines in the game of strength training; they are players in their own right. They play a crucial role in your body's adaptation to exercise, helping you get stronger, fitter, and healthier. So, as you continue your strength training routine, remember to balance work with rest and effort with recovery, creating a symphony of strength that plays to the rhythm of your body's needs.

And now that we've set the stage for a safe and effective strength training routine, we are ready to delve into the heart of strength training - the exercises. In the next chapter, we will explore an array of exercises suitable for seniors, providing you with the tools to build your strength training repertoire. So, let's keep the rhythm going, step by step, rep by rep, set by set, towards a stronger, healthier you.

4

AGE-FRIENDLY STRENGTH TRAINING CONCEPTS

Have you ever listened to a piece of music that was so predictable it became boring? Each note follows the last in such a regular pattern that you can anticipate the following note before it's played. Now, imagine that piece of music is your workout routine. Day after day, you perform the same exercises in the same order, with the same weights. Over time, this routine might become just as monotonous as the predictable piece of music, making you lose interest. But what if you could add some variation to your workout routine, just as a skilled musician adds variation to a piece of music to keep it interesting? This is where the concept of periodization comes in.

Periodization and Its Benefits

Periodization is a method of organizing your training into distinct periods, each with a specific goal. It's like a composer creating a symphony, with each movement contributing to the overall piece. In the context of strength training, these periods can focus on different aspects, such as building endurance, strength, or power.

Understanding Training Cycles

In an example of a periodized training program, a year can be divided into three cycles: macrocycle, mesocycle, and microcycle.

1. The macrocycle is the longest cycle, typically covering a year. This is like the complete symphony, encompassing all the different movements.
2. Mesocycles are shorter training periods within the macrocycle, typically lasting a few weeks to a few months. Each mesocycle can focus on a specific fitness component, like endurance, strength, or power. These are like the different movements in a symphony, each with its unique rhythm and tempo.
3. Endurance Phase: The emphasis is on high rep ranges (such as 15-20 reps) with shorter rest periods, using moderate to light weights. This phase improves muscular endurance and cardiovascular health.
4. Hypertrophy Phase: This phase aims to increase muscle size. The typical rep range is 8-12 reps with moderate rest periods. The tempo can vary, often involving a slower eccentric (lowering) phase to increase time under tension, a potential mechanism for muscle growth.
5. Strength Phase: The focus shifts to lifting heavier weights at a lower rep range (4-6 reps). Longer rest periods are allowed to enable full recovery between sets. The tempo can be more explosive to maximize strength gains.
6. Power Phase (if applicable): This phase involves very high-intensity, explosive movements at low reps, focusing on developing power.
7. Microcycles are the smallest training units, usually a week long. These are like the individual notes within a movement, each one contributing to the overall composition.

By adopting this systematic approach, you can ensure that different aspects of fitness are adequately addressed, reducing the risk of over-training and plateaus. Periodization also allows for recovery phases, which are essential for muscle growth and injury prevention. The variety in training can keep workouts interesting and challenging, increasing adherence and long-term success.

Periodization caters to the physical aspect of training and considers the psychological component, helping maintain motivation and focus. By progressing through different phases, you can continually challenge your body and adapt, leading to consistent improvements in strength, endurance, and muscle mass.

BENEFITS OF VARIED WORKOUTS

Just as a varied diet provides a range of nutrients, a varied workout program offers multiple benefits. It prevents your body from adapting too much to one type of stimulus, ensuring continued progress. It's like offering a varied menu to your muscles, keeping them engaged and responsive to the training.

Varied workouts can also help prevent overuse injuries that can occur from repeating the same movements too frequently. It's like playing different pieces of music on a piano to prevent wearing out the same keys.

Moreover, varied workouts can keep you mentally engaged, preventing boredom and maintaining motivation. It's like listening to a varied playlist, keeping your ears tuned and your mind interested.

Avoiding Plateaus

A common challenge in strength training is hitting a plateau, where progress seems to stall despite continued efforts. It's like a musician practicing the same piece over and over but not getting any better.

Periodization can help avoid this plateau effect. You can keep making progress by varying your workouts and continually challenging your body in new ways. It's like a musician adding new pieces to their repertoire, continually challenging their skills and avoiding stagnation. By systematically changing reps, weight, tempo, and exercises over time, you will stay engaged and motivated and see faster results.

Periodization can be a valuable tool in your strength training toolbox. By understanding its principles and benefits, you can create a varied, effective, and engaging workout program. Unfortunately, most people do not utilize or know about the concept of periodization, therefore not maximizing their progress and results with exercise. Later in this book, you will discover examples of beginner, intermediate, and advanced-level periodized strength training and opportunities for personalized strength training and coaching.

So, let's play our symphony of strength training with skill and variation, creating a masterpiece of fitness and health.

Progressive Overload for Seniors

Imagine yourself standing at the base of a gentle hill. At first, the incline is minimal, and you ascend with ease. Gradually, the hill becomes steeper, but your strength has grown with each step, allowing you to continue climbing. This is the principle of progressive overload, a key component of effective strength training.

Gradual Increase in Intensity

In the context of strength training, progressive overload refers to the gradual increase of stress placed on the body during exercise. It is the act of continuously challenging your muscles as they adapt and become stronger. For seniors embarking on a strength training program, applying the principle of progressive overload is crucial. However, it's equally important to ensure gradual and safe progression. Think of it as slowly adding weights to a scale. You wouldn't lift a heavy weight all at once but would instead add smaller weights over time, maintaining the balance and integrity of the scale.

Gradually increasing the intensity of your workouts could involve:

- Lifting heavier weights.
- Performing more repetitions of an exercise.
- Increasing the number of sets.
- Reducing the rest time between sets
- Performing a more challenging exercise variation

For instance, if you're comfortably performing two sets of ten repetitions with a certain weight, you might add a third set or increase the weight slightly.

Monitoring Your Progress

As you apply the principle of progressive overload, it's essential to keep track of your progress. This is comparable to marking the growth of a plant. By observing and keeping track of its height, you can appreciate how much it has grown and adjust your care accordingly.

In strength training, monitoring your progress involves keeping track of the weights you lift, the number of repetitions and sets you perform, and how these numbers increase over time. This can be done in a training log or a digital fitness tracker. Additionally, it's a wise decision to track the RPE (rate of perceived exertion) of each exercise. This is done by rating an exercise on a scale from 0 to 10, with 10 being the maximum effort. A good rule to follow is that most strengthening exercises should be around a 7 to 8 effort. This ensures you are challenging your body enough to adapt and get stronger but not overworking. It is acceptable to attempt a 9 or 10 effort level occasionally, but only after ensuring proper form, recovery, and confidence. Other times, it may be good to have a lighter recovery workout where intensity levels may only be a 5. By documenting your progress, you can see the fruits of your labor, which can be incredibly motivating. It also helps you plan your future workouts, knowing when and how to increase the intensity.

Adjusting Your Workout Over Time

The principle of progressive overload is not a one-time adjustment but rather a continuous process. As your body adapts to the current stress level, the workout that once challenged you may begin to feel easy. When this happens, it's time to adjust your workout again, increasing the intensity to continue challenging your muscles.

This is where your training log or fitness tracker comes in handy. By reviewing your documented progress, you can make informed decisions about how to adjust your workouts. Perhaps you're ready to lift a heavier weight, or maybe you can perform an extra set of your favorite exercises. It can also be very motivating to look back on previous training sessions to see your progress.

While it's important to keep challenging yourself, listening to your body is equally important. If you're experiencing excessive fatigue, persistent soreness, or any other discomfort, it may be a sign that you're pushing too hard. In such cases, scaling back a bit or allowing more recovery time may be beneficial. If you end up in a state of over-training, it will actually slow your progress and increase your risk of injury.

In essence, progressive overload is about walking the fine line between challenge and caution. It's about continuously pushing your boundaries while also respecting your limits. So, as you continue to climb your hill of strength training, remember to pace yourself, enjoy the journey, and celebrate each step of progress along the way.

VOLUME, LOAD, WEIGHT, REPS, AND TEMPO: GETTING THE BALANCE RIGHT

Understanding Volume

In the world of strength training, volume holds a pivotal role. Much like the volume control on your television, it determines the intensity of your experience. However, in strength training, volume controls the total amount of work you do in a workout instead of controlling the level of sound.

A simple way to understand volume is to picture a construction site where bricks are used to build a wall. Each brick represents a repetition, and the total number of bricks used daily represents the volume of work. If you lay 50 bricks one day and 100 bricks the next, your volume of work has increased.

As mentioned previously, in strength training, volume is calculated by multiplying the weight lifted (load) by the number of repetitions (reps) and the number of sets. For instance, if you perform 3 sets of 10 reps lifting a 5-pound weight, your total volume would be 150 pounds (3 sets x 10 reps x 5 pounds = 150 pounds). Again, your goal should be to increase volume over time gradually. In this example, the following week, you could obtain 165 pounds of volume (3 sets x 11 reps x 5 pounds = 165 lbs). This small change was just adding an additional repetition to each set. You could also either increase the sets or load to increase volume. It is typically not a good idea to attempt to alter more than one variable at a time, as this may lead to overtraining and increased injury risk.

Deciphering Load

Understanding load in strength training is like understanding the weight of each brick used in building a wall. The load refers to the amount of weight you're lifting or the resistance you're working against during an exercise.

Let's consider the bicep curl exercise. The dumbbell you lift represents the load. If you switch from a 5-pound dumbbell to a 10-pound dumbbell, you've increased the load. It's like you've switched from using lighter bricks to heavier ones in building your wall.

Adjusting the load is a key factor in tailoring your workout to your abilities and goals. If you're new to strength training, you might start with lighter loads and gradually increase as your strength improves.

Choosing the Right Weight

Selecting the appropriate weight is similar to choosing the right tools for a task. When it is too light, the task becomes too easy. When it is too heavy, the task becomes overly challenging and potentially unsafe.

In strength training, the right weight should challenge your muscles without compromising your form or causing discomfort. A good rule of thumb is to choose a weight that makes the last two to three repetitions of each set challenging but still doable with proper form.

The weight might be too light if you can easily complete all the reps without feeling challenged. On the other hand, if you can't complete the reps with proper form or you feel joint pain, the weight might be too heavy.

Remember, the goal here is not to lift the heaviest weights possible but to challenge your muscles safely and effectively. It's not about building the tallest wall in a day but about laying each brick with precision and care, creating a strong and sturdy structure over time.

Mastering Repetitions

Adjusting the number of repetitions in strength training is like tuning an instrument – too few, and you don't harness the full melody of your potential; too many, and you risk straining your body's harmony. In senior strength training, managing repetitions is crucial for steady progress, health maintenance, and injury prevention.

Initially, start with a repetition range that feels challenging yet manageable, such as around 8-12 reps. This range is effective for building strength without overburdening your muscles. The same number of repetitions that once felt challenging may become easier as you progress. This is a sign of your growing muscular strength and endurance.

When this occurs, it's time to modify your routine. You can increase the repetitions slightly, aiming for a range that challenges your muscles anew, such as 12-15 reps, yet still allows you to maintain good form throughout. This gradual increase ensures continuous muscle engagement and growth, adapting your body progressively to higher demands. It's about finding that sweet spot – enough repetitions to stimulate muscle growth and endurance, but not so many that your form falters or you experience joint discomfort.

Remember, the aim is not just to lift weights but to build a healthier, stronger you. Like a carefully composed symphony, each repetition is a note that contributes to the grander melody of your fitness and well-being. By thoughtfully adjusting your repetitions over time, you create a balanced and sustainable strength training routine that keeps you thriving in your senior years.

Exploring Tempo

Tempo in strength training for seniors is like the rhythm in music - each phase of the movement, whether concentric, eccentric, or isometric, contributes to the overall harmony of the exercise. Manipulating the tempo adds a layer of complexity and efficacy to your workouts, enhancing results, preventing injury, and refining form.

The concentric phase - when you lift, push, or push the weight - can be quickened to increase muscle power or slowed down to boost strength. A faster concentric phase recruits fast-twitch muscle fibers, essential for quick, powerful movements. Conversely, a slower lift increases time under tension, which can benefit stability, muscle growth, and endurance. An example of the shoulder press exercise's concentric phase is when pressing the dumbbell overhead.

The eccentric phase - when you lower the weight - is often overlooked but holds immense potential for strength gains. Slowing down this phase increases muscle control and emphasizes strength and stability. It helps absorb force, a key factor in injury prevention, and is especially important for seniors. Eccentric training can also improve joint stability and enhance flexibility. For the shoulder press exercise, the eccentric phase is when you lower the weight back down.

The isometric phase - where you hold the weight in a static position - is a test of endurance and control. This phase can be incorporated at any point in the movement – at the top, bottom, or mid-range – to challenge your muscles differently. Holding a position for a few seconds can help increase muscle activation and endurance. Isometrics can also be a valuable tool for pain management.

By manipulating these phases, you introduce new challenges and stimuli for your muscles. This variation not only accelerates results but also keeps the workouts engaging. Moreover, focusing on the tempo helps maintain proper form throughout the exercise, reducing the risk of injury.

Again, tempo variations are like fine-tuning your instrument - they bring precision, control, and efficiency to your strength training regimen. This approach allows for a comprehensive development of muscle function, contributing significantly to your overall health and mobility as a senior.

Understanding and adequately adjusting volume, load, weight, reps, and tempo are crucial in creating an effective and safe strength training routine. These elements are like the different instruments in a symphony, each playing a unique role. Only when they are balanced and harmonized can they create a beautiful piece of music. Similarly, balancing volume, load, and weight can help you create a strength training routine that is safe, effective, and tailored to your specific needs and goals.

Low-impact, High-Result Strength Training

Imagine you're at a beautiful beach, the warm sand beneath your feet, the gentle waves lapping at the shore. Now imagine these waves as your exercise routine. They are powerful, yes, but they're also gentle, causing no harm to the delicate sand structures on the beach. This is the essence of low-impact exercise—a powerful yet gentle way to improve your fitness. In this section, we'll explore the benefits of low-impact strength training, delve into some effective options, and discuss how this approach can help protect your joints.

Benefits of Low-Impact Exercise

Low-impact exercises are those that place minimal stress on your joints. This can be beneficial in situations when joint pain or irritation is present. Picture a gentle stream flowing over pebbles. The water shapes and smooths the pebbles over time but doesn't damage them. Similarly, low-impact exercises strengthen your muscles over time while placing lower forces on your joints.

A primary benefit of low-impact exercise is that it allows you to exercise safely, potentially reducing the risk of injury. This particularly benefits seniors with joint issues or other age-related conditions that make high-impact exercises challenging.

Low-impact exercises can aid in improving your balance and coordination, crucial factors in preventing falls and maintaining independence as you age. They also enhance general cardiovascular health and promote weight management, contributing to overall health and well-being.

It's like a gentle yet powerful force, steadily sculpting your body, enhancing your strength, and boosting your health without causing harm or discomfort.

Low-Impact Strength Training Options

There is a wide array of low-impact exercises that can be incorporated into your strength training routine. They're like the different strokes in a painting, each contributing to the overall masterpiece.

One such strengthening exercise is the seated leg press. As you push against the resistance, your leg muscles engage and strengthen, all while you're comfortably seated, without high-impact forces being placed on your joints, such as with running or jumping.

Another excellent low-impact upper-body strength training exercise is the seated row. Using a resistance band or a rowing machine, this exercise targets your upper body muscles, enhancing strength and improving posture without placing undue stress on your joints.

Resistance bands, in general, are an excellent tool for low-impact strength training. They provide resistance that challenges your muscles, but their flexibility and versatility allow for a range of joint-friendly exercises. Bands are also a great tool to have at home or when traveling to help stay consistent with a strength training routine.

Additional Low-Impact Strength Training Exercises:

- Wall Push-Ups: Ideal for those who find traditional push-ups too challenging. Standing at arm's length from a wall and pushing against it works the chest, shoulders, and arms.

- Chair Squats: Perfect for leg and lower body strength, these involve sitting and standing from a chair, ensuring minimal stress on the knees.
- Pilates: Focuses on core strength, flexibility, and overall muscle toning through controlled movements, which is beneficial for balance and stability.
- Tai Chi: This martial art emphasizes slow, controlled movements, enhancing flexibility, balance, and strength in a low-impact manner.
- Aquatic Exercises: Activities like water aerobics or swimming provide resistance for muscle strengthening while the buoyancy of water reduces stress on joints.
- Step-Ups: Using a low step or bench, stepping up and down strengthens leg muscles without the high impact of traditional jumping or running.

Low-Impact Strength Training Activities:

- Yoga: Strength-focused yoga styles (like Vinyasa or Hatha) can build muscle strength and flexibility with minimal joint impact.
- Cycling: Stationary or outdoor cycling is excellent for building leg strength and cardiovascular fitness without harsh impact on the knees.
- Elliptical Training: This machine offers a cardiovascular workout that mimics running but with less impact on joints.
- Walking with Hand Weights: A brisk walk combined with light hand weights can effectively tone the upper body while providing a low-impact cardio workout.

Incorporating a variety of these exercises and activities into a strength training routine can offer seniors a balanced approach to fitness, focusing on muscle strength, flexibility, and joint health.

Remember, the key is to choose exercises that you enjoy, and that suits your abilities, ensuring you can maintain the routine in the long run. The long-term goal is to find strengthening exercises that are challenging, feel comfortable, and do not produce pain. It's like choosing your favorite songs for a playlist – you're likelier to listen to it regularly if it includes the songs you love.

Protecting Your Joints

Joint protection is paramount in any strength training routine, particularly for seniors. It's like a protective layer of bubble wrap around a fragile item, safeguarding it from damage.

Low-impact exercises inherently protect your joints by minimizing the stress placed on them. However, other strategies can further enhance joint protection.

One such strategy is maintaining proper form during exercise. Proper form ensures that the right muscles are doing the work and that your joints are moving in a safe and effective manner. Think of it as a carefully choreographed dance, where each movement is precise and controlled, ensuring a beautiful performance while preventing missteps.

Another strategy is to incorporate flexibility and balance exercises into your routine. Flexibility exercises, such as stretching, can help maintain a good range of motion in your muscles and joints. In contrast, balance exercises can improve your stability and prevent falls, protecting your joints from injury.

In addition, regular rest and recovery can help protect your joints. Rest periods allow your joints to recover from the stress of exercise, reducing the risk of overuse injuries.

However, our bodies and joints are designed to be very durable and adaptable. As you get stronger, you may find that certain positions or exercises that were once challenging or caused discomfort no longer do. This, in part, is because your body adapted, creating stronger muscles, bones, and joints to tolerate force.

To sum up, low-impact, high-result strength training is a gentle yet effective way to enhance your strength, improve your fitness, and protect your joints. With various exercises to choose from and multiple strategies to safeguard your joints, it's a method that is beneficial but also enjoyable and sustainable. So, let's embrace this gentle wave of exercise, allowing it to shape and strengthen us and carry us toward the shore of health and well-being.

As we close this chapter, we carry the knowledge and tools to create a safe and effective strength training routine. We understand the importance of periodization and progressive overload, we know how to balance volume, load, and weight, and we're ready to embrace low-impact strength training. With these tools in hand, we're well-equipped to continue exploring strength training, discover the exercises that will form the core of our routine, and put our knowledge into action. So, let's keep the rhythm going, step by step, rep by rep, set by set, towards a stronger, healthier you.

BUILDING YOUR AT-HOME STRENGTH TRAINING GYM: EQUIPMENT ESSENTIALS

P icture yourself in a bustling, crowded gym. The clamor of weights clanging, the continuous hum of treadmills, the loud music echoing through the speakers. Now, imagine a serene, peaceful room in your home. The quiet is calming, and the environment is familiar. Which scenario seems more inviting? If you're leaning towards the tranquility of your home, you're not alone. Many seniors prefer the comfort and convenience of working out at home or even a combination of at-home and fitness center exercise routines. The good news is that building an at-home gym for strength training doesn't require a colossal investment or a lot of space. It's more about selecting the right tools that offer versatility, safety, and effectiveness for your workouts.

EQUIPMENT RECOMMENDATIONS

Adjustable Dumbbells

Consider adjustable dumbbells as your versatile companions in strength training. With the simple turn of a dial or change of a plate, you can alter the weight you're lifting, making it lighter or heavier based on your current strength level. They are like multiple dumbbells rolled into one, saving you space and providing a range of weight options. A good standard adjustable dumbbell set may range from 5 to 50 pounds, giving you plenty of resistance from shoulder to lower body exercises.

Resistance Bands

Next, imagine resistance bands as your flexible friends. They can add an element of resistance to a wide variety of strength training exercises. The beauty of resistance bands lies in their simplicity - they're lightweight, easy to store, and can be used for a whole host of exercises, from bicep curls to overhead shoulder presses. In addition, bands are very budget-friendly and easy to travel with.

Stability Ball

Consider the stability ball as a fun yet challenging addition to your at-home gym. While it might look like an oversized beach ball, don't be fooled by its innocent appearance. It's an incredibly effective tool for enhancing balance, stability, and core strength. You can use it for exercises like wall squats or even as a dynamic replacement for your chair during seated exercises.

Yoga Mat

A yoga mat might seem like a humble piece of equipment, but its value is immense. It provides a comfortable, non-slip surface for your workouts, protecting your joints during floor exercises. Like a dedicated space for your strength training routine, it subtly signals your brain that it's time to focus and work out.

Ankle Weights

Ankle weights are a compact tool that can provide excellent resistance with various exercises. These can be placed around your ankles, knees, or even wrists. Examples of possible exercises include side-lying leg raises or even a bicep curl (great modification for those with wrist or finger pain).

5

Adjustable Weight Bench

While not a necessity, an adjustable weight bench can be a versatile addition to your at-home gym. Picture it as a chameleon of sorts, adapting to serve various purposes. It can be set at an inclined position for chest presses, flat for seated exercises, or even used as a support for step-ups. However, if space or budget is a concern, don't worry. Most exercises performed on a bench can also be modified to be performed on a mat or with the support of a sturdy chair.

And finally, remember that your own body can be utilized as a great source of resistance for strength training. Using your body against gravity is functional and attainable for anyone to include. The exercise options are endless, from bodyweight squats and push-ups to standing calf raises.

Selecting the right equipment for your at-home gym is like choosing the right ingredients for a recipe. Each one plays a unique role, contributing to a successful workout, much like each ingredient contributes to a delicious meal. With these tools at your disposal, you're well-equipped to indulge in effective, safe, and enjoyable strength training workouts right in the comfort of your home.

SPACE SETUP AND SAFETY MEASURES

Setting up your home gym is similar to organizing your personal workspace. Just as you would ensure a desk is at the right height or your chair is comfortable for those long hours of work, similar attention to detail is required when establishing your workout area. Here's how you can create a safe and functional space for your at-home strength training routine:

Adequate Lighting

The first pointer on our checklist is lighting. Proper illumination is crucial for maintaining visual acuity during your workouts. Good lighting will help you see clearly, ensuring you can perform exercises with the correct form and avoid any potential hazards. Think of it as having a well-lit stage for a performance. The spotlight allows the performer to move with certainty without worrying about missteps.

Similarly, a well-lit workout space will enable you to exercise with confidence. On another note, poor lighting is a common cause of falls in seniors. By ensuring your workout area and home have adequate lighting, you can help decrease your risk of falling.

Non-Slip Flooring

Next, let's shift our focus to the flooring. When engaging in strength training, a stable footing is absolutely vital. Therefore, consider investing in non-slip mats or installing non-slip flooring. This will provide you with a sturdy surface to perform your exercises and reduce the risk of slips or falls. It's equivalent to wearing a pair of good running shoes while jogging - they provide the necessary traction, keeping you steady on your feet. Another option is wearing athletic shoes that have good grip and traction. The last thing you want is to wear socks on tile or wood floors, which is an easy way to slip and fall.

Clearing Space of Obstacles

Now, take a moment to scan your workout area for any potential obstacles. These could be furniture, loose rugs, or random objects lying around. Clearing these items will create a more spacious and safer environment for your workouts. It's like removing pebbles off a running track, ensuring a smooth, uninterrupted run. A decluttered space means you can focus solely on your workout without worrying about bumping into something.

Proper Ventilation

Just as plants need a regular supply of fresh air for growth, your body needs fresh air when working out. Proper ventilation in your workout space ensures a steady supply of fresh air, making breathing easier and helping you stay comfortable, especially during those intense workout sessions. So, ensure there are enough sources of fresh air, like windows, or consider using a fan or an air purifier to improve the air quality.

Emergency Contact Information

Finally, safety is always important. In case of emergencies, it's essential to have the necessary contact information at your fingertips. Keep your phone within reach during your workouts and have essential numbers - like that of a family member, friend, or your doctor - saved on speed dial. Think of it as a safety net, there to catch you if and when you need it.

With these safety measures in place, you're all set to enjoy a safe and efficient workout from the comfort of your home. As you build strength, remember that every step of this process - from setting up your workout space to performing each rep and set - contributes to your overall progress. So, here's to creating a safe, effective, and enjoyable at-home gym for strength training.

EXAMPLES OF EFFECTIVE AT-HOME EXERCISES

Chair Squats

Imagine the simple act of sitting down and standing up from a chair. This everyday movement is, in essence, a squat - a functional exercise that strengthens your lower body and enhances balance. A chair can be a great tool to support you as you familiarize yourself with this exercise, providing stability and helping you maintain proper form.

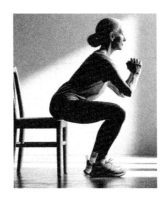

To perform:

1. Stand in front of a sturdy chair with your feet hip width apart.
2. Keep your chest up and your back straight.
3. Slowly lower your body as if you were sitting down until your hips touch the chair.
4. Pause for a moment.
5. Push through your heels to stand back up.
6. This completes one repetition.

Remember to ensure that your entire foot maintains contact with the ground, not favoring only your heels or forefoot.

Wall Push-ups

If traditional push-ups seem intimidating, wall push-ups are an excellent alternative. They target the same muscles - the chest, shoulders, and arms - but with less strain on the wrists and shoulders.

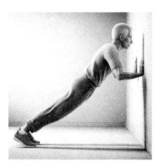

To perform this exercise:

1. Stand facing a wall, about an arm's length away.
2. Place your hands on the wall at shoulder height, slightly wider than shoulder-width apart.
3. Keeping your body straight, bend your elbows to bring your chest towards the wall.

4. Press your hands into the wall to push your body back to the starting position.

This completes one repetition.

Seated Leg Lifts

Seated leg lifts are a gentle exercise that can help strengthen your thigh muscles. All you need is a sturdy chair to sit on.

To perform:

1. Sit down on a chair or a comfortable surface.
2. Straighten one leg out in front of you.
3. Hold the leg in this position for a couple of seconds.
4. Slowly lower your leg back down in a controlled manner.
5. Try to keep your leg from dropping down quickly.
6. Repeat the movement on one side several times before switching to the other leg.

Standing Leg Curls

Standing leg curls are great for targeting the muscles at the back of your thighs - your hamstrings. They can be performed using just your body weight, with ankle weights, or a resistance band for added challenge.

To Perform:

1. Stand behind a chair, holding onto it for support.
2. Slowly bend one knee, lifting your heel towards your buttocks.
3. Lower your foot back down in a controlled manner. This completes one repetition.
4. Perform the entire set on one leg, then switch to the other leg.

Seated Resistance Band Row

The seated resistance band row is a versatile exercise that targets your upper back and arms, promoting good posture and upper body strength.

To perform:

1. Sit on a chair.
2. Place a resistance band under both feet.
3. Hold the ends of the band with your hands.
4. Keeping your back straight, pull the band towards your waist.
5. Squeeze your shoulder blades together.
6. Slowly release the band to return to the starting position.
7. This completes one repetition.

Step Ups

Step-ups are an effective exercise that targets your lower body and helps enhance your balance and coordination. This exercise imitates the motion of climbing stairs, a simple day-to-day activity that people often overlook.

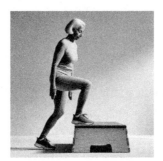

To perform:

1. Stand in front of a sturdy step or low platform, feet shoulder-width apart.

2. Place your right foot on the step, ensuring your entire foot is on the surface.
3. Press through your right foot to lift your body up, bringing your left foot to meet the right on the step.
4. Pause briefly at the top, then step down with the left foot, followed by the right. This completes one repetition.
5. Focus on keeping your back straight and your movements controlled throughout the exercise.

To increase the intensity, you can add weight or increase the height of the step.

Plank

The Plank is a powerful exercise for strengthening your core, which includes the muscles around your trunk and pelvis. It's a foundational pose in many fitness routines, offering a full-body workout focusing on stability.

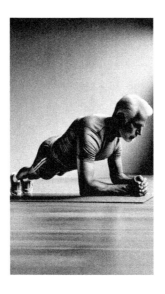

To perform:

1. Start by lying face down on the floor.

2. Rise onto your elbows and toes, keeping your elbows directly under your shoulders and your body in a straight line from head to heels.

3. Engage your core, thighs, and glutes to maintain the position.

4. Ensure your back doesn't sag and your hips don't lift too high.

5. Hold this position for a set duration, starting with shorter intervals and gradually increasing as you build strength.

6. Modify by placing your elbows on a bed or couch instead of the floor.

Bird Dog

The bird dog is an excellent exercise for improving balance and core strength. It targets the abdominals, lower back, glutes, and thighs and enhances coordination and stability.

To perform:

1. Begin on your hands and knees, with your hands directly under your shoulders and knees under your hips.

2. Keeping your back flat and gaze down, slowly extend your right arm forward and left leg back, creating a straight line from your extended hand to your foot.

3. Hold this position for a few seconds, then return to the starting position.

4. Repeat with the left arm and right leg. This completes one repetition.

5. Keep your movements slow and controlled, focusing on balance and stability.

6. Modify by only lifting your arm or leg individually.

Incorporating some of these exercises into your strength training routine can provide a solid foundation for enhancing strength, balance, and overall fitness. We will dive into more possible exercises in the next chapter and in your 4-week training program at the end of this book. Remember, the focus is on quality, not quantity. Performing each exercise with proper form and control is far more beneficial than rushing through a large number of repetitions. So, take your time, enjoy the process, and watch your strength and confidence grow with each rep and set.

STRENGTH TRAINING WITH HOUSEHOLD ITEMS

Soup Can Bicep Curls

Let's start with a simple and familiar item - soup cans. They can be excellent makeshift weights for bicep curls.- Stand tall with a soup can in each hand, arms fully extended, and palms facing forward.

1. Keep your elbows close to your body.
2. Flex your elbows and curl the cans towards your shoulders.
3. Pause momentarily.
4. Slowly lower your arms back to the starting position

Congratulations, you've just performed a bicep curl! Aim for 10-15 repetitions to start with, maintaining a slow, controlled motion throughout.

Water Bottle Arm Raises

Next, grab a couple of water bottles. These can serve as light weights for arm raises, which target the shoulders.

- Stand or sit upright.
- Hold a water bottle in each hand, arms by your sides, and palms facing inward.
- With a controlled movement, raise your arms to the sides until they're at shoulder level.
- Lower them back down.

Remember, it's not a race. The slower and more controlled the movement, the more effective the exercise.

Chair Dips

A sturdy chair can be an excellent prop for dips, an exercise that targets the tricep muscles in your upper arms.

1. Sit on the edge of the chair, hands gripping the edge next to your hips.
2. Walk your feet out in front of you.
3. Keeping your back close to the chair, lower your body towards the floor by bending your elbows.
4. Push yourself back up to the starting position to complete one repetition.
5. Aim to perform around 10-15 repetitions, keeping your movements slow and controlled.

Laundry Detergent Deadlifts

Let's consider your laundry detergent bottle. Its handle provides an easy grip, and its weight can be suitable for deadlifts, a compound exercise that works multiple muscle groups.

1. Stand tall, holding your laundry detergent bottle with both hands in front of your thighs.
2. Hinge forward at your hips, allowing the detergent bottle to lower towards the floor while keeping your back straight.
3. Drive through your feet to stand back up.
4. Squeeze your glutes at the top.

Repeat this movement for 10-15 repetitions.

Milk Jug Rows

A full 1-gallon milk jug can provide great resistance for this back exercise. While standing, gently lean forward while keeping your back flat. You can place one hand on a chair for support while the other hand holds the milk jug. Perform a row, pull the milk jog to your chest, and then control it back down. Repeat for 10-15 repetitions to start.

As you can see, strength training doesn't require fancy gym equipment. Everyday household items can be repurposed into practical fitness tools, allowing you to engage in strength training right in the comfort of your home. With these exercises, you're well-equipped to continue your strength training routine, even on days when you can't make it to the gym or prefer to stay home.

So, go ahead and give these exercises a try. They're proof that when it comes to fitness, sometimes the simplest tools can be the most effective. With a bit of creativity and a commitment to your health, you can turn everyday items into your personal gym equipment, proving that strength training is not just accessible but also adaptable to your lifestyle.

And remember, each rep, each set, and each workout contributes to your overall progress. So, whether you're lifting dumbbells in a gym or soup cans at home, know that every bit of effort counts. You're not just building muscle; you're building a healthier, stronger, and more vibrant version of yourself. So, let's keep going, growing, and glowing, one rep, one set, one workout at a time.

And now, as we set down our laundry detergent bottles and take a moment to appreciate our progress, let's look forward to the next chapter of our strength training exploration. We will continue to explore detailed instructions and helpful tips for exercises tailored to seniors. So, prepare to learn, move, and strengthen as we continue our strength training adventure.

UNLOCK THE POWER OF GENEROSITY

"Kindness is a language which the deaf can hear and the blind can see." - Mark Twain

People who give selflessly tend to live more prosperous, more fulfilling lives. And if there's a chance to spread that joy in our journey, well, I'm all in.

So, here's a heartfelt request...

Would you extend a helping hand to someone you've never met without expecting anything in return?

Who is this mystery person, you wonder? They're a lot like you. As seniors seek to improve their health and wellness, they often require guidance.

Our goal is simple: to make the benefits of Strength Training for Seniors known to everyone. But to truly make an impact, I need to reach... everyone.

This is where your kindness shines. People often choose a book based on its cover and, importantly, its reviews. So, on behalf of a senior who's just starting their strength training journey, I humbly ask:

Would you leave a review for this book?

It's a gift that costs nothing but a minute of your time, yet it can profoundly impact another senior's life. Your review could be the key that unlocks...

...a healthier lifestyle for another senior.
...increased mobility and independence for a grandparent.
...improved strength and balance for a friend.
...enhanced well-being for a community member.
...a journey of transformation for someone just like you.

To share your kindness and truly make a difference, all it takes is less than 60 seconds to...leave a review.

Just scan the QR code below or click here to share your thoughts:

If the thought of helping an unseen friend warms your heart, then you're absolutely my kind of person. Welcome to our community of caring individuals. You're one of us now.

I can't wait to guide you through the effective and safe strength training techniques that can enhance your life as a senior. The tips and strategies in the upcoming chapters are sure to excite you.

Thank you sincerely for your generosity. Let's continue our journey to a stronger, healthier life together.

Your biggest fan, Rush Hemphill PT, DPT, CSCS

PS - Remember, sharing valuable knowledge increases your value in the eyes of others. If you believe this book can help another senior in your life, please pass it on. Let's spread strength and health together!

6

CUSTOMIZED STRENGTH EXERCISES FOR SENIORS

Imagine the excitement of a child in a toy store, eyes wide with awe and wonder, surrounded by an array of colorful toys. Each toy offers a unique form of engagement, be it a puzzle that challenges the mind, a ball that encourages physical activity, or a doll that sparks creativity. Now, replace those toys with exercises, and you have a similar scenario in strength training. Each exercise offers unique benefits, be it boosting energy, improving balance, enhancing joint health, or challenging different fitness levels.

In this chapter, we will explore a diverse range of exercises, each designed to meet your specific needs as a senior. Like a child in a toy store, you have the freedom to choose the exercises that resonate with you and align with your fitness goals. So, let's step into this exercise toy store and discover the vibrant array of options that await us.

EXERCISES TO BOOST ENERGY AND WARM UP

Energy is the fuel that powers all of our daily activities, from cooking and playing with grandchildren to tending to the garden. Here are some simple exercises that are designed to boost your energy levels and keep you feeling active and vibrant throughout the day. These are just a few examples that can be easily performed at home.

Marching in Place

Marching in place is a simple yet effective exercise to get your heart pumping and energy flowing. It's like being in a parade, marking time to the beat of your own drum. Stand tall, engage your core, and lift your knees, alternating between right and left. You can increase the intensity by swinging your arms or lifting your knees higher. Aim for 1-2 minutes of marching to start, gradually increasing as your stamina improves.

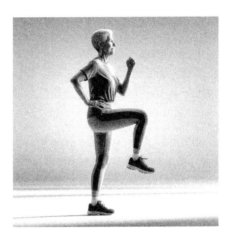

Seated Jumping Jacks

Seated jumping jacks offer all the cardiovascular benefits of traditional jumping jacks without the impact on your joints. It's like watching a movie from the comfort of your couch rather than a crowded cinema; you get the same enjoyment but with added comfort and less stress. Sit on the edge of a sturdy chair, engage your core, and mimic the movements of a standing jumping jack by alternating between opening and closing your arms and legs. Start with performing 1 minute of work, increasing as your endurance improves.

Arm Circles

Arm circles are an excellent exercise to warm up your shoulders and upper body. Imagine drawing circles in the sky with each hand, feeling the energy radiate from your shoulders down to your fingertips. Extend your arms out to the sides and perform small circular movements, first in a forward direction, then backward. Aim for 10-20 circles in each direction, adjusting the size or speed of the circles for more or less intensity.

Seated Bicycle Crunches

Seated bicycle crunches are a low-impact exercise that engages your core, enhances circulation, and kicks your energy levels up a notch. It's like pedaling a bicycle, only you're seated comfortably on a chair. Sit on the edge of a chair, lean back slightly, and place your hands behind your head. Bring one knee towards your chest and twist your torso to meet your opposite elbow to your knee. Alternate sides in a pedaling motion, aiming for 10-15 reps on each side.

These energy-boosting exercises are like your morning cup of coffee, providing a jolt of energy to kickstart your day. Remember, the goal isn't speed but rather consistency and enjoyment. So, take your time, listen to your body, and let the rhythm of these exercises infuse your day with energy and vitality.

Exercises to Improve Balance

Maintaining balance is akin to walking a tightrope. It requires a keen sense of body awareness, strength in the right places, and a focus that doesn't waver. As we age, maintaining this balance can become increasingly challenging. However, the good news is that with targeted exercises, we can significantly improve our balance, reduce the risk of falls, and enhance our overall mobility. So, let's put on our metaphorical balancing shoes and explore these exercises.

Heel-to-Toe Walk

Think of a fashion model strutting down the runway, one foot directly in front of the other. The heel-to-toe walk is a similar exercise. It's easy to do, requires no equipment, and effectively improves balance.

Start by standing tall and looking straight ahead. Place one foot in front of the other so that the heel of your front foot touches the toes of your back foot. Take a step, placing your weight on your heel, then shift your weight forward to your toes. Repeat this sequence for 15-20 steps to start. This exercise can be modified and made easier by placing your feet farther apart. This will give you slightly more stability if needed when starting out. To make it more challenging, try performing with your eyes closed.

Standing Single-Leg Balance

Imagine a flamingo standing tall on one leg, the embodiment of grace and balance. The single-leg stand is an exercise that mimics this elegant bird's stance.

Begin by standing straight. Slowly lift one foot off the ground, keeping your leg aligned with your body. Maintain this position for as long as comfortable, then switch to the other leg. As your balance improves, challenge yourself by extending the duration of the stand or by closing your eyes. A good goal is to be able to balance for at least 10 seconds on each leg.

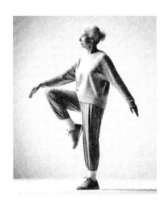

Heel Raises

Picture a ballet dancer gracefully rising onto her tiptoes. The heel raise, or calf raise, is an exercise that encapsulates this graceful movement, working your calf muscles and enhancing your balance.

Stand straight with your feet hip-width apart. Slowly raise your heels off the ground, shifting your weight onto your toes. Lower your heels back down in a controlled manner. Repeat this movement for 10-15 repetitions. If needed, you can hold onto a wall or counter slightly for balance.

Toe Lifts

Now, let's reverse the heel raise movement with toe lifts. This exercise strengthens your shin muscle, also known as your tibialis anterior, a lesser-known but important muscle group for balance and walking.

While standing, keep your heels firmly on the ground and lift your toes as high as you can. Hold this position for a moment, then lower your toes back to the ground. Aim for 10-15 repetitions. Again, you can hold onto the wall or a counter for added balance.

Tandem Stance

To perform this exercise, start by standing with one foot in front of the other, placing your heel to toe. Try to maintain your balance in this position for up to one minute. If you want to increase the difficulty level, you can cross your arms or even close your eyes. If you need additional support, you can modify the exercise by holding onto a chair, counter, or wall. Aim for 30-60 seconds each side.

Tai Chi Movements

Tai Chi, an ancient Chinese martial art, is often described as "meditation in motion." It combines deep breathing with flowing movements, improving balance, flexibility, and peace of mind.

There are several Tai Chi movements that can enhance balance, such as "Parting the Wild Horse's Mane" or "Grasping the Bird's Tail." Although it's best to learn Tai Chi from a qualified instructor, there

are many online resources available to guide you through the movements.

Incorporating these balance exercises into your routine can significantly enhance your stability, reduce fall risk, and improve overall mobility. Remember, just like a tightrope walker doesn't perfect his skill overnight, improving balance takes time and practice. So, be patient with yourself, celebrate your progress, and, most importantly, enjoy the process.

Balance is not about perfection but about embracing the wobbles and teetering moments, knowing that with each one, you're becoming stronger, steadier, and more confident. So, keep practicing, improving, and balancing one exercise, one rep, one set at a time.

JOINT-FRIENDLY EXERCISE OPTIONS

Caring for your joints is akin to maintaining a well-oiled machine. Regular movement, combined with specific joint-friendly exercises, keeps the machine running smoothly and efficiently. However, it's crucial to choose exercises that promote joint health without causing undue stress or strain. Let's explore some joint-friendly exercise options that can be easily incorporated into your fitness regimen.

Water Aerobics

Picture a calm, serene pool. The water is warm and inviting, providing a buoyant environment that's gentle on your joints. This is the setting for water aerobics, a low-impact exercise that offers a full-body workout. The water's buoyancy supports your weight, reducing stress on your joints, while its resistance challenges your muscles, providing a balanced and effective workout.

Water aerobics classes often include a variety of exercises, from marching and jogging to leg lifts and arm curls, all performed in the water. The movements are smooth and fluid, much like the water itself, promoting joint mobility and flexibility. Picture yourself moving rhythmically to the beat of music, the water gently resisting your movements, providing a gentle yet effective workout.

Chair Yoga

Now, let's transition from the buoyant environment of the pool to the comfort of a chair with chair yoga, a modified version of traditional yoga that makes the practice accessible to those with mobility issues. Just as a sturdy tree adapts its branches to reach toward the sunlight, chair yoga adapts traditional yoga poses for practice on a chair, making it an excellent exercise option for seniors.

Chair yoga incorporates a variety of stretches and poses designed to promote flexibility, strength, and balance, all performed from the comfort of a chair. Picture yourself seated comfortably, stretching your arms towards the sky, then gently twisting your torso, each movement guided by your breath. This practice not only benefits your physical health but also promotes relaxation and mental calm, making it a holistic exercise option.

Pilates

Pilates, much like yoga, is a mind-body exercise that emphasizes core strength, flexibility, and body awareness. It does so using a series of controlled movements and specific breathing techniques. Picture a conductor leading an orchestra, each movement deliberate and controlled, contributing to a beautiful symphony. Pilates mirrors this precision and control with its controlled movements and focus on body awareness.

Many Pilates exercises can be modified to be performed either seated or lying down, reducing strain on your joints. Another popular version is wall pilates, which is geared towards many seniors. The movements are slow and controlled, focusing on quality rather than quantity, making Pilates a safe and effective exercise option for seniors.

Low-Impact Cardio

Finally, let's step onto the path of low-impact cardio. These exercises get your heart pumping, improving cardiovascular health without jarring your joints. Consider activities like brisk walking, cycling on a stationary bike, or even dancing. Each of these activities increases your heart rate, promoting cardiovascular health, without the high-impact stress that activities like running or jumping can place on your joints.

Low-impact cardio exercises can be easily adjusted to match your fitness level. For instance, you can increase your walking pace, add resistance on the stationary bike, or include more vigorous dance moves as your fitness improves. Picture yourself on a nature walk, your pace brisk and your heart pumping, or cycling on a stationary bike, your favorite music playing in the background, your legs pedaling in rhythm with the beat.

Incorporating these joint-friendly exercises into your fitness routine can significantly enhance your joint health, overall mobility, and quality of life. Remember, joint health is not a destination but an ongoing process, much like maintaining a well-oiled machine. With regular movement and these specific exercises, you can keep your machine - your body - running smoothly and efficiently, promoting longevity and a vibrant, active lifestyle.

So, whether you're floating in a pool, seated on a chair, or striding confidently on a path, know that each movement and each exercise is a step towards better joint health and overall well-being. Enjoy the process, listen to your body, and most importantly, keep moving.

CATERING TO VARIOUS FITNESS LEVELS

Beginner: Seated Exercises

Starting your strength training journey from the comfort of a chair can be a great way to build confidence and lay a strong foundation for more advanced exercises. Here are some examples of beginner-friendly exercises that you can perform while seated:

Seated Leg Extensions:

Seated leg extensions are an effective way to strengthen your quadriceps, the muscles at the front of your thighs.

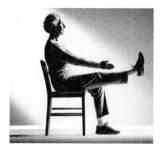

1. Start by sitting tall on a chair, feet flat on the ground.
2. Extend one leg out straight, hold for a moment, and then slowly lower it back down.
3. Repeat this motion for 10-15 repetitions before switching to the other leg.

As you become stronger, you can add ankle weights for added challenge and resistance.

Seated Overhead Press:

The seated overhead press is an exercise that focuses on strengthening your shoulder muscles. It can be performed with light weights or even household items such as soup cans.

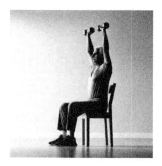

1. Hold your weights at shoulder level.
2. Slowly push them up toward the ceiling until your arms are fully extended.
3. Lower them back down to shoulder level to complete one repetition.

4. Repeat the process for 10-15 times.

Seated Marching

This is a great exercise to strengthen your hip flexors and core muscles. Add ankle weights to increase intensity.

To perform:

- Sit upright in a sturdy chair
- Lift one leg up, bringing your knee toward your chest
- Control your leg back down, and repeat on the other side
- Continue for 30-60 seconds

Intermediate: Standing Exercises

Once you've mastered the seated exercises and feel ready for a new challenge, it's time to move on to standing exercises. These exercises offer a greater range of motion, require more balance and stability, and engage more muscles, providing a more comprehensive workout. You can use a sturdy chair or wall for support as you perform these exercises. Remember, there are endless exercises and variations. These are just a few of my favorites that are effective and offer multiple benefits.

Standing Knee Lifts/Marching:

Knee lifts are a great way to strengthen your hip flexors and improve balance.

1. Hold onto a chair for support.
2. Stand tall.
3. Slowly lift one knee up towards your chest.
4. Lower it back down and repeat.
5. Aim for 15-20 repetitions on each leg.
6. Add ankle weights to increase intensity.

Standing Calf Raises:

This is an excellent exercise for strengthening your calf muscles and ankles.

1. Stand on the ground with your feet flat.
2. Press through your toes and lift your heels up as high as you can.
3. Pause for one second at the top.
4. Return to the starting position.

To increase the intensity, you can perform it off a step or stair to increase the range of motion. If needed, hold onto a chair or wall for support.

Wall Push-Ups:

Wall push-ups are a great way to strengthen your upper body without straining your wrists.

1. Stand an arm's length away from a wall.
2. Place your palms on the wall.
3. Bend your elbows to bring your chest towards the wall.
4. Push back to the starting position to complete one rep.
5. Aim for 10-15 repetitions.

Once this becomes relatively easy, progress to more challenging variations, such as push-ups on the floor.

Standing 1-Arm Shoulder Press:

This exercise improves your balance, core strength, and shoulder muscles.

1. Stand and hold a dumbbell by one shoulder using one hand.
2. Raise the dumbbell overhead.
3. Pause for a moment when the dumbbell is at the top.
4. Slowly lower the dumbbell back down.
5. Complete 10-15 repetitions on one side.

Switch to the other side and repeat the same process.

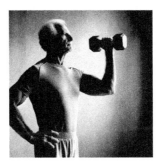

Advanced Exercises

As your strength and confidence grow, you should be ready to tackle more challenging exercises. These exercise variations will target multiple muscle groups simultaneously, offering a time-efficient way to enhance your overall strength.

Squats:

Squats are an effective exercise that targets your entire lower body. You can progress to standing squats once you feel comfortable with basic chair squats. To do this:

- Stand with your feet hip-width apart.
- Bend your hips and knees as if sitting back in a chair.
- Push through your feet to stand back up and aim for 10-15 repetitions.
- To maintain adequate balance and stability, keep your entire foot in contact with the ground throughout the exercise.
- For an added challenge, hold weights in your hands to increase the load and further your strength gains.

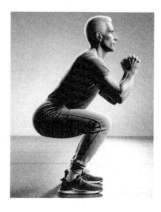

Reverse Lunges:

Lunges are another excellent lower-body exercise with several different variations. A reverse lunge is an easier variation to start with and more knee-friendly than a forward lunge.

1. Begin in a standing position.
2. Take a step backward with one foot.
3. Lower your body until both knees are bent around a 90-degree angle. Modify by not going as low or increase difficulty by going lower.
4. Push through your front foot to return to standing.
5. Repeat the exercise on the other side.
6. Aim for 10-15 repetitions per leg.
7. To increase the intensity, hold weights in your hands while performing the exercise.

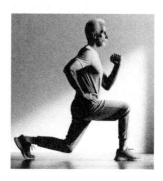

Standing Rows:

Standing rows target your upper body, specifically your back muscles.

1. Stand with your feet hip-width apart
2. Hold a resistance band or cable machine with both hands
3. Extend your arms straight out in front of you
4. Pull your elbows back, squeezing your shoulder blades together
5. Aim for 10-15 repetitions

Shoulder Tap Push-ups:

This is a challenging variation of push-ups that emphasizes shoulder and core stability. To perform this exercise:

- Start with a regular push-up, then lift one hand up and touch the opposite shoulder at the top.
- Keep your trunk and hips steady, and focus on moving only your shoulder and arm.
- Return your hand to the floor and perform another push-up, then repeat the same movement on the opposite shoulder.
- Start with ten reps and gradually increase over time. If you find it difficult, you can modify the exercise by performing push-ups with your hands on a chair, table, or wall.

Deadlifts:

The deadlift is a fundamental movement pattern that you use throughout your life. Whenever you lift something off the floor, you're performing a variation of a deadlift movement. This full-body exercise targets your hips, back, core, and grip strength. If you're new to this exercise, start with a kettlebell and then progress to a trap bar or barbell as you become more comfortable with the movement.

To perform a deadlift with a kettlebell:

1. **Starting Position:** Stand with your feet hip-width apart, with the kettlebell placed between your feet. Your feet should be pointed slightly outward.

2. **Grip and Posture:** Bend at your hips and knees to squat down and grip the kettlebell. Your back should be flat, not rounded, to protect your spine. Your shoulders should be back, and your chest should be up, looking forward.

3. **Lifting the Weight:** Engage your core and keep your back straight as you lift the kettlebell off the ground. Drive through your feet, bringing your hips forward and standing up straight. The motion should come from your hips and legs rather than your back. The kettlebell should remain close to your body as you lift.

4. **Top Position:** At the top of the lift, your legs should be straight, and your shoulders should be back. Squeeze your glutes at the top of the movement for full hip extension.

5. **Lowering the Weight:** To lower the kettlebell back to the ground, hinge at your hips and push your buttocks back. Keep your back straight and lower the weight along the same path it came up, keeping it close to your body. Bend your knees once the kettlebell passes them.

6. **Repeat:** Allow the kettlebell to touch the ground lightly before performing the next repetition. Keep your movements controlled and steady.

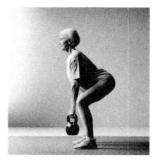

Start with a lighter weight to master the form before progressing to heavier weights like a trap bar or barbell. Consider consulting with a fitness professional to ensure your technique is correct and safe.

Embracing the diversity of strength training exercises can help keep your workouts exciting and challenging. Whether you're just starting with seated exercises, advancing to standing exercises, or tackling full-body workouts, each step you take is a testament to your progress. By choosing exercises that suit your fitness level and challenge you safely and effectively, you can ensure that your strength training routine is beneficial, enjoyable, and sustainable. So, let's continue exploring, experimenting, and exercising, one rep, one set, one workout at a time.

In this chapter, we have explored a broad spectrum of exercises, each designed to cater to different needs and fitness levels. As we journey through the world of strength training, remember that there's no one-size-fits-all approach. Each person's journey is unique, and what matters most is finding the exercises that fit your abilities, meet your needs, and bring joy to your routine. So, whether you're lifting weights, balancing on one leg, or performing a seated leg extension, know that each movement, each effort, is a step towards a stronger, healthier, and more vibrant you. As we turn the page to the next chapter, let's carry forward this spirit of exploration and individuality, ready to delve even deeper into the world of strength training for seniors.

7

OVERCOMING COMMON STRENGTH TRAINING CHALLENGES

Strength training for seniors, like any worthwhile endeavor, comes with its own set of challenges. From the fear of injury to managing muscle soreness, sticking to the routine, and progressing workout intensity, these challenges can sometimes seem like steep hills on your fitness path. However, these hills can be transformed into vantage points with the right strategies, offering you a better view of your strength and resilience. In this chapter, we will explore these challenges and equip you with practical solutions to navigate them effectively.

ADDRESSING FEAR OF INJURY

The fear of injury is a common concern among seniors when starting a strength training routine. It's akin to walking in an unfamiliar neighborhood, where every corner feels uncertain. However, you can navigate this new path confidently and safely with the right approach.

Proper Form and Technique

Maintaining proper form and technique while strength training is crucial to achieving desired results. Proper form ensures that the right muscles are engaged during each exercise and reduces the risk of injury. For instance, when doing a squat, keeping your knees in line with your feet can help prevent unnecessary strain on your knees.

If you're new to strength training, consider working with a fitness professional or physical therapist to learn the correct form for each exercise. They can provide personalized instruction and feedback, helping you master the techniques. Think of them as seasoned guides who will show you the ropes in this new terrain.

Importance of Warm-ups and Cool-downs

Warm-ups and cool-downs are the opening and closing acts of your strength training performance. They prepare your body for the workout and help it recover afterward, reducing the risk of injuries.

Before you start strength training, spend 5-10 minutes doing light cardio exercises such as walking, cycling, elliptical, or marching in place. This warm-up phase gradually increases your heart rate, warms up your muscles, and lubricates your joints, preparing your body for the workout. It's like tuning an instrument before a performance, setting the stage for a harmonious symphony.

After your workout, spend another 5-10 minutes cooling down. This can involve slow walking or gentle stretching exercises. The cool-down phase helps your heart rate and breathing return to normal and reduces muscle stiffness. It's akin to the calm after the storm, returning your body to its state of rest.

Listening to Your Body

When navigating the path of strength training, your body is your compass, providing valuable feedback through various signals. Listening to this feedback is crucial to prevent injuries and ensure your workout is effective.

Pay attention to how your body feels during and after each workout. If you experience pain, dizziness, or excessive shortness of breath during an exercise, it's a signal to stop and rest. Similarly, feeling excessively fatigued or sore for more than 48 hours after a workout might indicate that you've pushed too hard and need more recovery time.

Remember, it's not about competing with others or pushing beyond your limits. It's about exercising within your capacity and gradually increasing your strength. It's like walking at a comfortable pace, not racing to keep up with others.

Regular Rest Days

In the symphony of strength training, rest days are the pauses between the notes, providing much-needed recovery time for your body. These pauses are as critical as the notes in creating a beautiful melody.

Regular rest days in your workout routine give your muscles time to repair and strengthen themselves. It can also help prevent overuse injuries that can occur from exercising the same muscle groups too frequently.

A good rule of thumb is to have at least one rest day between strength training sessions. These rest days can include light activities such as easy aerobic exercise, walking, or stretching, which keep your body active without overly stressing your muscles.

Addressing any fear of injury can involve:

- Learning proper form and technique.
- Warming up and cooling down appropriately.
- Listening to your body's signals.
- Incorporating regular rest days

With these strategies, you can turn the unfamiliar neighborhood of strength training into a well-trodden path where each step is confident, safe, and effective.

MANAGING MUSCLE SORENESS AND FATIGUE

Engaging in strength training can sometimes lead to muscle soreness and fatigue. It's akin to feeling the burn after a long trek, a sign of your muscles working hard and adapting to new challenges. Here are some strategies to manage muscle soreness and fatigue effectively.

Hydration and Nutrition

Staying hydrated and fueling your body with the proper nutrients is like watering a plant and providing it with the appropriate soil nutrients - it's fundamental for growth and recovery.

Drinking plenty of water, aiming for about 8-10 glasses (approximately 2-2.5 liters) daily, helps flush out toxins from your body and keeps your muscles hydrated, reducing soreness. It's like a soothing bath, washing away the day's dust and grime. Aim to drink water before, during, and after your workouts and throughout the day to maintain adequate hydration levels.

Nutrition is essential for muscle recovery. A balanced combination of proteins, carbohydrates, and healthy fats provides the energy required to perform and recover from workouts. Think of it as a balanced diet for your muscles, providing all the necessary nutrients for growth and repair. Include lean proteins, whole grains, fruits, and vegetables in your meals, and consider having a protein-rich snack after your workout to aid muscle recovery.

Rest and Recovery

Rest and recovery are like the silent portions of a music track, allowing you to catch your breath before the next note strikes. During rest periods, your body works to repair and strengthen the muscles worked during exercise, reducing soreness and fatigue.

Ensure you're getting enough sleep, as it is during this time that most repair and recovery processes occur. Sleep is like a peaceful interlude, allowing your body to refresh and rejuvenate for the next day.

Also, incorporate active rest days between your workout sessions. These rest days can involve light activities like walking or stretching, which keep you active without stressing your muscles. Think of it as a peaceful stroll between intense races, allowing your body to recover and prepare for the next challenge.

Stretching

Gentle stretching after your workouts can help alleviate muscle soreness. It's like a gentle cool-down walk after a race, helping your body transition from a state of high activity to rest.

Focus on stretching the muscle groups you worked on during your exercise session. Hold each stretch for about 30 seconds, ensuring that it does not bounce or force the stretch. It's all about gentle, sustained stretches that help increase flexibility and reduce muscle tension.

Heat and Cold Therapy

Applying heat or cold to sore muscles can provide temporary relief and speed up recovery, but it's essential to understand when and how to use each method effectively.

Cold therapy, such as applying ice packs, may be beneficial immediately after exercise or an injury. Some research suggests that cold therapy helps reduce muscle soreness and inflammation by constricting blood vessels, which decreases blood flow to the area. This method, akin to a refreshing splash of cold water, is instantly cooling and soothing. It's especially effective for acute injuries or pain, swelling, and inflammation. The cold can also numb the sore tissue, acting as a local anesthetic. However, it's important to avoid cold therapy if you have circulatory or sensory disorders, as it can exacerbate these conditions. In addition, cold therapy should not be over-utilized or relied upon. Only incorporate if absolutely needed to decrease muscle soreness or short-term pain. In the long term, your body is designed to heal and repair on its own.

Heat therapy can be beneficial for chronic muscle pain or stiffness. It works by increasing blood flow and circulation to the affected area and can be administered through warm baths or heating pads. This increase in blood flow brings more oxygen and nutrients to the muscles, helping to heal damaged tissue. It's a comforting, warm hug to your muscles, soothing and healing simultaneously. Heat therapy is particularly beneficial before exercise to increase muscle flexibility and decrease stiffness. However, it should not be used immediately after an injury, as it might increase inflammation and swelling. It's also advisable to avoid heat therapy if you have diabetes, dermatitis, vascular diseases, deep vein thrombosis, or an open wound.

When using either therapy, it's crucial to protect your skin. Wrap ice packs or heat pads in a towel before applying to prevent direct contact with the skin. Also, limit each application to 15-20 minutes to prevent skin damage. Do not use heat or cold therapy if the skin sensation is impaired, such as in cases of neuropathy.

Managing muscle soreness and fatigue involves more than staying hydrated and nourished, getting enough rest and recovery, and stretching gently. Integrating heat or cold therapy as part of your routine can significantly aid in muscle recovery. However, understanding when to use each type of therapy and following safety guidelines ensures that these methods are both effective and safe, preparing you for the next step in your strength training routine.

STICKING TO YOUR WORKOUT ROUTINE

Setting Realistic Goals

In the grand tapestry of your strength training routine, each stitch represents a goal - an intention that guides your actions. However, the key to effective goal-setting lies in being realistic. Picture a lighthouse standing tall amidst a vast ocean. Its light is visible and reachable, guiding the sailors safely to shore. Similarly, realistic goals are like your personal lighthouses, providing a visible, reachable target to guide your efforts.

Realistic goals consider your current fitness level, health conditions, and personal circumstances. For instance, if you're new to strength training, a realistic goal might be to complete two 20-minute sessions per week. As your strength and stamina improve, you can adjust your goal, aiming for three sessions per week or gradually increasing the duration of each session.

Remember, the aim is not to immediately reach for the stars but to build a sturdy ladder, one rung at a time. With each goal met, you climb one rung higher, edging closer to your ultimate fitness aspirations.

Creating a Schedule

With your goals set, the next step is to create a schedule for your workouts. A well-planned schedule is like a roadmap, outlining the path towards your destination - your fitness goals. It provides structure to your routine, ensuring you allocate adequate time for your workouts amidst your daily responsibilities.

When creating your workout schedule, consider your lifestyle and daily routine. Find the time of day when you feel most energetic and can focus on your workout without distractions. For some, this might be early morning; for others, it could be late afternoon.

Also, remember to schedule rest days between your workout sessions. These rest days are like the empty spaces in a piece of music, providing balance and aiding recovery.

With a well-planned schedule, your strength training routine can become an integral part of your lifestyle, like a steady beat in the rhythm of your day.

Variety in Workouts

Adding variety to your workouts is like adding different colors to a painting. It not only makes the routine more exciting but also enhances its effectiveness. Different exercises target different muscle groups, ensuring a balanced and comprehensive workout.

For instance, one day, you could focus on upper body exercises like push-ups, bicep curls, and overhead presses. The next session could be dedicated to lower-body exercises like squats and lunges. You could also incorporate balance exercises or flexibility stretches into your routine.

Variety keeps you mentally engaged and motivated, making your workout routine more enjoyable. It's like sampling different dishes at a buffet, each bringing its unique flavor and appeal.

Celebrating Progress

In the midst of your strength training routine, it's important to pause and appreciate the progress you've made. Each milestone achieved, no matter how small, is a testament to your efforts and deserves to be celebrated.

This could be lifting a heavier weight, performing an extra set, or noticing improvements in your daily activities, like easily climbing stairs or carrying groceries without feeling winded. These improvements are like shining stars in the night sky, each a beacon of your progress.

Remember, progress is not just about the destination but also the journey. Each step forward, each milestone achieved, brings you closer to your fitness goals, painting a larger picture of health, strength, and vitality.

Sticking to your workout routine is an ongoing process shaped by realistic goals, a well-planned schedule, variety in workouts, and regular celebration of progress. With these strategies, you can weave an effective, enjoyable, and sustainable routine. Each stitch and thread contributes to the grand tapestry of your fitness journey, creating a masterpiece of strength, health, and vitality.

PROGRESSING YOUR STRENGTH TRAINING

Gradual Increase in Intensity

Envision yourself tuning a musical instrument. You wouldn't yank the tuning pegs. Instead, you'd turn them gradually, tightening the strings bit by bit until you reach the perfect pitch. Similarly, progressing your strength training involves a slow and steady increase in intensity, avoiding abrupt changes that might lead to injury or burnout.

This progression can take several forms. It could be adding more repetitions to your sets or lifting a slightly heavier weight. Maybe it's reducing the rest time between sets, or it could be performing a more challenging version of an exercise. The key is to make these increases gradually, giving your body time to adapt and grow stronger.

Incorporating New Exercises

Think of your strength training routine as a recipe you're perfecting. While you may start with a basic set of ingredients (exercises), over time, you might want to add in some new flavors. Incorporating new exercises into your routine not only targets different muscle groups but also adds variety, keeping your workouts interesting and engaging.

When introducing a new exercise, start with a lighter weight or a smaller range of motion if needed, gradually increasing as your comfort and proficiency improve. Whether it's a new resistance band exercise, a stability ball workout, or a balance challenge, each new addition brings a fresh dimension to your strength training routine, enhancing its effectiveness and appeal.

Challenging Balance and Coordination

Imagine a tightrope walker high above the ground. Every step requires balance and coordination, every movement precise and controlled. While strength training might not involve such risky feats, improving balance and coordination is integral to the process.

Exercises that challenge your balance and coordination enhance your physical skills and stimulate your brain, promoting cognitive health. It could be a single-leg stand, a stability ball exercise, or a yoga pose. These exercises add an element of challenge to your routine, pushing you to improve and grow physically and mentally stronger.

Regular Fitness Assessments

Consider a gardener monitoring the growth of the plants. Regular checks help assess the plants' health, spot any signs of disease early, and make necessary adjustments to their care. Similarly, regular fitness assessments are crucial to track your strength training progression.

These assessments help track your progress, identify areas of improvement, set goals, and guide future workout plans. It could be as simple as noting down the weights you lift, the repetitions you perform, or how your body feels during and after workouts. Or it could involve more formal assessments like strength, flexibility, or balance tests. Here are a few examples of fitness assessments you can test and track over time:

1. 30-second sit-to-stand: Start by sitting in a standard, sturdy chair. Set a timer for 30 seconds, and perform as many squats up and back down to the chair as possible, making sure to stand all the way up.
2. Single leg balance: Set a timer, then balance on one leg for as long as you can. Repeat on the other side.
3. Push-ups (wall push-ups, modified push-ups, and full push-ups). First, determine which variation is most suitable for you. Perform as many repetitions as you can. As your strength improves, consider testing a harder variation.
4. 6-minute walk test: Set a timer for 6 minutes, then walk as fast and far as you can in 6 minutes. Take note of how far you went. Ideally, this is performed on an indoor or outdoor track so you can easily track your distance. Consider taking your heart rate before and after the walk to asses your cardiovascular response.

Regularly checking your progress makes you more attuned to your body, understanding its strengths, and recognizing its potential. It's a way of celebrating your achievements while inspiring you to keep moving forward.

In strength training, progression is not a sprint but a marathon. It's about moving forward at the right pace for you, celebrating each milestone, and continually striving for improvement. Whether increasing your workout intensity, adding new exercises, challenging your balance, or assessing your fitness, each step forward is a testament to your strength, resilience, and determination. So, as you continue your strength training routine, remember to be patient with yourself, to listen to your body, and to enjoy the process. After all, strength training is not just about physical strength but also about the inner strength that comes from overcoming challenges, embracing change, and persisting in the face of adversity.

As this chapter comes to a close, let's carry these insights forward, ready to face challenges, embrace progression, and continue on the path to improved strength and vitality. The next chapter awaits, ready to further guide us on this exciting path of strength training for seniors.

8

FUELING YOUR STRENGTH: NUTRITION ESSENTIALS FOR SENIORS

I magine standing in a vast, colorful market brimming with fresh produce, lean meats, whole grains, and a multitude of other nutritious foods. The air is filled with the aroma of ripe fruits, fresh vegetables, and warm bread. This is your nutrition market; each food item symbolizes a nutrient that fuels your strength training journey.

Understanding the importance of quality ingredients in a gourmet recipe is like understanding the role of nutrition in strength training. The quality of the ingredients determines the dish's taste and nutritional value, just as the quality of your nutrition influences the effectiveness of your strength training.

NUTRITION BASICS FOR SENIORS

The Role of Nutrition in Strength Training

Strength training is a physical activity that involves the breakdown of muscle fibers. When you lift weights or do other types of strength training exercises, your muscles undergo microscopic tears and damage. This process is similar to a sculptor chipping away at a block of marble to create a statue. In order to repair and strengthen your muscles, your body needs essential nutrients such as protein, carbohydrates, and fats. These nutrients act like a sculptor's chisel and mallet, making your muscles stronger and more defined.

Balancing Your Macros: Understanding Proteins, Carbohydrates, and Fats

Macronutrients, commonly known as macros, are the nutrients your body requires in large amounts: proteins, carbohydrates, and fats. Each of these plays a crucial role in fueling and supporting your strength training routine, contributing to both your performance and recovery.

Proteins: Often referred to as the building blocks of muscles, proteins are essential for the repair, growth, and maintenance of muscle tissue. During strength training, muscle fibers undergo stress and micro-tears. Protein facilitates the repair and rebuilding of these fibers, leading to muscle growth and increased strength. High-quality protein sources include lean meats like chicken and turkey, fish rich in omega-3 fatty acids like salmon and tuna, eggs, and dairy products like Greek yogurt and cottage cheese. Lentils, beans, tofu, tempeh, and quinoa are excellent choices for plant-based options. The amino acids found in protein-rich foods are crucial for muscle recovery, especially after intense workouts.

Carbohydrates: Carbohydrates are the primary energy source for your workouts. They are broken down into glucose, which fuels your muscles for physical activity. Consuming adequate carbohydrates ensures that you have enough energy to perform at your best during strength training sessions. Whole grains, such as brown rice, quinoa, and whole wheat, provide sustained energy release, while fruits and vegetables offer not only quick energy but also essential vitamins and minerals for overall health. It's important to include a variety of carbohydrate sources in your diet to ensure a balanced intake of nutrients.

Fats: Often misunderstood, fats play a vital role in overall health and exercise performance. They serve as a long-term energy source, particularly useful during prolonged or lower-intensity exercise. Fats are also essential for absorbing fat-soluble vitamins (A, D, E, and K), which are crucial for many bodily functions, including bone health and immune function. Sources of healthy fats include avocados, nuts and seeds, olive oil, and fatty fish. Incorporating these into your diet helps ensure your body has the necessary energy reserves and supports optimal health.

Each macronutrient has a unique and vital role in supporting your strength training. Proteins repair and build muscle, carbohydrates provide the energy needed for your workouts, and fats offer a reserve fuel source while aiding in nutrient absorption. A balanced diet that adequately supplies these macronutrients is essential for optimal performance in strength training and overall physical health.

Protein Requirements

Proteins are the building blocks of your muscles, crucial for their repair, growth, and maintenance. For seniors, especially those engaged in strength training, consuming adequate protein is like providing the necessary bricks to construct a sturdy wall. According to the Academy of Nutrition and Dietetics, active seniors typically need more protein than their less active counterparts - about 1.2 to 1.5 grams per kilogram of body weight per day. This increased intake supports muscle repair, growth, and overall recovery following exercise.

A varied and balanced diet rich in high-quality protein sources is key to meeting these increased protein needs. Here's a list of high-protein foods that can be incorporated into your diet:

- **Meat:** Chicken breast, turkey, lean beef, and pork are excellent sources of high-quality protein.
- **Fish:** Fatty fish like salmon and tuna provide protein and beneficial omega-3 fatty acids.
- **Eggs:** Highly versatile and rich in protein, eggs are one of the most bioavailable sources of protein.

- **Dairy:** Milk, cheese, Greek yogurt, and cottage cheese offer a good balance of protein and other essential nutrients.
- **Legumes:** Beans, lentils, and chickpeas are great plant-based protein sources.
- **Nuts and Seeds:** Almonds, walnuts, flaxseeds, and chia seeds provide protein along with healthy fats.
- **Tofu and Tempeh:** Protein options for those following a vegetarian or vegan diet.
- **Protein Supplements:** Whey or plant-based protein powders can be a convenient way to boost protein intake, especially post-workout.
- **Protein Bars:** A handy and quick source of protein, ideal for snacking, especially when on the go.

By incorporating a variety of these protein-rich foods into your diet, you can ensure that your body receives the necessary nutrients to support your strength training efforts. Remember, it's not just about the quantity of protein consumed but also the quality and the combination of different protein sources that make a balanced diet.

Importance of Fiber

Dietary fiber is like a street cleaner for your digestive system, helping to keep it clean and functioning smoothly. It adds bulk to your diet, helping you feel full and satisfied. Additionally, fiber supports heart health by helping to reduce cholesterol levels. Fruits, vegetables, whole grains, and legumes are all excellent sources of fiber.

Healthy Fats

Healthy fats, particularly omega-3 fatty acids, are like a protective shield for your heart. They help lower levels of bad cholesterol, reducing the risk of heart disease. Fatty fish like salmon, as well as flaxseeds, chia seeds, and walnuts, are rich in these heart-healthy fats.

Dietary Supplements: When Are They Needed?

Dietary supplements are like a backup generator. They can fill in nutritional gaps when your diet doesn't provide all the nutrients you

need. However, they are not a replacement for a balanced diet. Before starting any dietary supplement, it's important to consult with a healthcare provider or a registered dietitian.

Eating for Energy: Timing Your Meals Around Workouts

Eating before and after your strength training workouts is like topping up your car's gas tank before and after a long drive. A small, balanced meal or snack before training can provide energy for your workout. After training, another balanced meal or snack can provide nutrients for muscle recovery.

Overcoming Common Nutritional Challenges for Seniors

Nutritional challenges for seniors may include decreased appetite, difficulty chewing or swallowing, or limited access to fresh foods. Solutions may involve:

- Eating smaller, more frequent meals.
- Choosing soft or liquid foods.
- Utilizing meal delivery services.
- Consuming prepared foods

Support from healthcare professionals, such as a registered dietitian, can also be invaluable in overcoming these challenges.

In essence, nutrition is a critical component of your strength training routine. By understanding the role of nutrition and learning how to balance your macros, you can fuel your workouts effectively, support muscle recovery, and enhance your overall health. It's about choosing the right ingredients from your nutrition market and using them to create a gourmet recipe for strength training success.

Role of Hydration in Strength Training

Consider the analogy of a well-oiled machine operating smoothly and efficiently. The oil in this analogy represents water in our bodies, playing a crucial role in various physiological processes, including muscle contraction, nutrient transport, and temperature regulation. When we engage in strength training, our bodies require additional water to support these processes and ensure optimal performance.

Water Intake Guidelines

The amount of water each person needs can vary depending on numerous factors such as age, gender, weight, and activity level. However, a general guideline is to aim for at least eight glasses of water daily. This target increases when you engage in activities like strength training.

During a strength training session, our bodies lose water through sweat. To compensate for this loss, it is recommended to drink about 500ml of water 2-3 hours before your workout and then continue to sip on water throughout the session to stay adequately hydrated.

It's important to note that hydration isn't only about water. Beverages such as milk, juice, and herbal teas can also contribute to your daily fluid intake. Foods with high water content, such as fruits and vegetables, can also aid in maintaining hydration.

Signs of Dehydration

Dehydration can be compared to a warning light on a car's dashboard, indicating something is amiss. When we are dehydrated, our bodies send out signals, alerting us to the need for hydration.

Common signs of dehydration include a dry or sticky mouth, fatigue, headache, dizziness, and little or no urination. More severe symptoms can include rapid heartbeat, rapid breathing, and fainting.

Moreover, studies suggest that even mild dehydration can impair physical performance, mood, and cognitive function, underscoring the importance of staying adequately hydrated, particularly during strength training.

Hydration and Muscle Recovery

Water plays a vital role in muscle recovery following a strength training session. Picture a construction site where bricks are being laid to build a wall. The bricks represent the proteins and amino acids that repair and build muscles, while the water represents the mortar that holds the bricks together. Without the mortar, the bricks would be loose and unstable. Similarly, without adequate hydration, muscle recovery and growth would be compromised.

Water helps transport nutrients to your muscles, aiding in their recovery and growth post-workout. Additionally, staying hydrated helps prevent muscle cramps and lubricates the joints, reducing the risk of injuries.

In essence, hydration is a key ingredient in the recipe for successful strength training. By adhering to water intake guidelines, recognizing the signs of dehydration, and understanding the role of hydration in muscle recovery, you can ensure that your strength training routine is well-supported and effective. So, as you lift those weights and strengthen those muscles, remember to lift that water bottle as well, replenishing your body one sip at a time.

VITAMINS, MINERALS, AND THEIR IMPORTANCE

Vitamin D and Bone Health

Let's begin by vividly picturing a bright, sunny day. The sunlight streaming down not only lifts your spirits but is also a primary source of Vitamin D. Often referred to as the 'sunshine vitamin,' Vitamin D plays an instrumental role in the maintenance of bone health, a factor of paramount importance in your strength training regimen.

Vitamin D aids in the absorption of calcium, a mineral crucial for bone strength and structure. It is as if Vitamin D is the key that unlocks the door, allowing calcium to enter and fortify the bones. This is particularly important for seniors, as bones can become more fragile and prone to fractures with age.

Strength training stimulates bone growth, and having adequate Vitamin D levels helps ensure that the calcium necessary for this growth is available. It is like having a well-stocked pantry when you decide to bake - all the necessary ingredients are at hand, ensuring a successful outcome.

Fatty fish like salmon and mackerel, fortified dairy products, and egg yolks are rich dietary sources of Vitamin D. However, due to limited food sources and reduced skin synthesis, seniors may struggle to get enough Vitamin D from sunlight and diet alone. In such cases, supplementation might be necessary following a consultation with a healthcare provider.

Calcium for Muscle Function

Shifting focus, imagine a well-rehearsed orchestra where each musician plays their part in perfect harmony, resulting in a beautiful symphony. In the symphony of our body, calcium can be likened to the conductor, playing a crucial role in muscle function.

Calcium is involved in the process of muscle contraction. It's as if calcium gives the starting signal, setting in motion the series of events that lead to a muscle fiber contracting. Therefore, having sufficient calcium is crucial for optimal muscle function during strength training.

Calcium is also essential for maintaining strong bones and teeth. Although dairy products are the most well-known sources of calcium, they can also be found in other foods like leafy green vegetables, fortified plant-based milks, and certain types of fish such as sardines and salmon. A balanced diet can help ensure adequate calcium intake. A healthcare provider might recommend taking a calcium supplement in case of insufficient dietary intake.

Iron and Energy Levels

Lastly, imagine a bustling city at peak hour, with traffic flowing smoothly along the extensive network of roads. In the bustling city of our body, iron acts like a transport system, carrying oxygen from the lungs to the muscles and facilitating the production of energy needed for strength training.

Iron is a key element of hemoglobin, a substance found in red blood cells that is responsible for carrying oxygen throughout the body. Insufficient levels of iron in the body can lead to reduced oxygen transport, which can cause fatigue and decreased physical performance. Therefore, it is essential for seniors who engage in strength training to maintain adequate iron levels to ensure optimal health and performance.

Iron-rich foods include lean meats, poultry, and fish. Plant-based sources include lentils, beans, and fortified cereals. Pairing these foods with a source of Vitamin C, such as citrus fruits or bell peppers, can enhance iron absorption. As with Vitamin D and calcium, a healthcare provider may recommend an iron supplement if dietary intake is inadequate.

All in all, ensuring an adequate intake of these key vitamins and minerals - Vitamin D, calcium, and iron - can support your strength training efforts, promoting bone health, muscle function, and energy production. It's like fine-tuning your instrument before a performance, setting the stage for a successful and effective workout. Remember, each note, each rhythm, and each rest in your strength training symphony plays a crucial role. So, focus on each one, and enjoy the beautiful music you're creating, one nutritious meal, one workout, one day at a time.

MEAL PLANNING AND PREPARATION TIPS

Batch Cooking

Imagine a well-stocked freezer filled with ready-to-eat meals. These aren't your average store-bought frozen dinners but wholesome, nutritious meals that you have prepared yourself. This is the beauty of batch cooking, also referred to as meal prepping," a time and energy-saving method that aligns perfectly with your strength training regimen.

Batch cooking is like tending to a garden where you sow seeds once but reap the benefits over time. You invest a few hours once or twice a week to prepare multiple meals, saving you time and effort on busier days.

To get started, select a few recipes that you enjoy and that align with your nutritional needs. Consider meals that freeze and reheat well, such as soups, stews, or casseroles. Next, make a shopping list and set aside time for cooking. Prepare your meals, portion them into individual containers, and freeze them. Now, you have a freezer full of nutritious meals, ready to fuel your body whenever needed.

Healthy Snack Ideas

With a bit of planning, you can have an arsenal of nutritious snack options at your disposal. Think of these healthy snacks as pit stops on your strength training journey, providing vital refueling to keep you going.

Protein-rich snacks like Greek yogurt, cottage cheese, or a handful of nuts can help repair and build muscles after a workout. Fresh fruits and vegetables paired with hummus or nut butter offer a mix of fiber, vitamins, and healthy fats. Whole-grain crackers with cheese or avocado provide a balanced combination of carbohydrates and protein.

Remember, the key is to plan ahead. Stock your kitchen with these healthy snack options so that when hunger strikes, you're prepared.

Reading Food Labels

Navigating the supermarket aisles can sometimes feel like deciphering a foreign language, with food labels sporting a jumble of nutritional information. However, understanding food labels can empower you to make informed choices, aligning your diet with your strength training goals.

Food labels contain a wealth of information, much like a book with a captivating story. The nutrition facts panel tells you the amount of proteins, carbohydrates, fats, and fiber in a serving of the product. It also gives information about the calorie content, helping you manage your energy intake.

The ingredients list reveals what exactly goes into the product. Ingredients are listed in descending order by weight, so the first few ingredients make up the largest portion of the product. Look out for whole foods at the beginning of the list, and be wary of long, unpronounce-able words, which often indicate the presence of artificial additives.

Reading and understanding food labels is like having a compass in the nutrition market, guiding you towards wholesome, nutritious choices that support your strength training efforts.

SAMPLE 7-DAY MEAL PLAN:

Here is an example of a 7-day meal plan for seniors, complete with macronutrient balance. Keep in mind that individual dietary needs may vary, so adjustments may be necessary based on your individual needs. This is not medical advice, so always consult a healthcare provider or registered dietician for specific nutrition advice based on your needs and medical history.

Day 1

Breakfast: Scrambled Eggs with Spinach and Whole Grain Toast

- Ingredients: 2 eggs, 1 cup of fresh spinach, 2 slices of whole grain bread, 1 tsp olive oil
- Macronutrients: Protein: 20g | Carbs: 30g | Fats: 15g

Lunch: Grilled Chicken Salad with Mixed Greens and Quinoa

- Ingredients: 100g grilled chicken breast, 2 cups mixed greens, ½ cup cooked quinoa, cherry tomatoes, cucumber, 1 tbsp balsamic vinaigrette
- Macronutrients: Protein: 30g | Carbs: 35g | Fats: 10g

Snack: Greek Yogurt with Berries and Almonds

- Ingredients: 1 cup Greek yogurt, ½ cup mixed berries, 10 almonds
- Macronutrients: Protein: 20g | Carbs: 20g | Fats: 10g

Dinner: Baked Salmon with Steamed Broccoli and Sweet Potato

- Ingredients: 150g salmon fillet, 1 cup broccoli, 1 medium sweet potato
- Macronutrients: Protein: 35g | Carbs: 40g | Fats: 20g

Total Daily Macronutrients: Protein: 105g | Carbs: 125g | Fats: 55g | Calories: 1415

Day 2

Breakfast: Oatmeal with Sliced Banana and Walnuts

- Ingredients: 1 cup cooked oatmeal, 1 banana, 1/4 cup walnuts
- Macronutrients: Protein: 10g | Carbs: 45g | Fats: 15g

Lunch: Turkey and Cheese Sandwich with Side Salad

- Ingredients: 2 slices whole grain bread, 100g sliced turkey breast, 1 slice cheese, mixed greens, cherry tomatoes, cucumber, 1 tbsp olive oil
- Macronutrients: Protein: 25g | Carbs: 40g | Fats: 12g

Snack: Cottage Cheese with Pineapple

- Ingredients: 1 cup cottage cheese, 1/2 cup chopped pineapple
- Macronutrients: Protein: 15g | Carbs: 20g | Fats: 2g

Dinner: Grilled Shrimp, Brown Rice, and Steamed Asparagus

- Ingredients: 150g shrimp, 1 cup cooked brown rice, 1 cup asparagus
- Macronutrients: Protein: 30g | Carbs: 45g | Fats: 8g

Total Daily Macronutrients: Protein: 80g | Carbs: 150g | Fats: 37g | Calories: 1253

Day 3

Breakfast: Whole Grain Pancakes with Greek Yogurt and Strawberries

- Ingredients: 2 whole grain pancakes, 1/2 cup Greek yogurt, 1/2 cup strawberries
- Macronutrients: Protein: 15g | Carbs: 50g | Fats: 10g

Lunch: Lentil Soup and Whole Grain Bread

- Ingredients: 1 cup lentil soup, 1 slice whole grain bread
- Macronutrients: Protein: 18g | Carbs: 40g | Fats: 5g

Snack: Apple Slices with Almond Butter

- Ingredients: 1 medium apple, 2 tbsp almond butter
- Macronutrients: Protein: 4g | Carbs: 25g | Fats: 18g

Dinner: Baked Chicken Breast with Quinoa Salad

- Ingredients: 150g chicken breast, 1/2 cup cooked quinoa, mixed vegetables (tomatoes, cucumber, bell pepper)
- Macronutrients: Protein: 35g | Carbs: 35g | Fats: 10g

Total Daily Macronutrients: Protein: 72g | Carbs: 150g | Fats: 43g | Calories: 1275

Day 4

Breakfast: Scrambled Tofu with Spinach, Mushrooms, and Whole Grain Toast

- Ingredients: 1/2 cup tofu, 1 cup spinach, 1/2 cup mushrooms, 1 slice whole grain toast
- Macronutrients: Protein: 20g | Carbs: 30g | Fats: 12g

Lunch: Tuna Salad on Mixed Greens

- Ingredients: 100g canned tuna, mixed greens, olive oil dressing
- Macronutrients: Protein: 25g | Carbs: 10g | Fats: 15g

Snack: Hummus with Carrot and Cucumber Sticks

- Ingredients: 1/4 cup hummus, 1 carrot, 1/2 cucumber
- Macronutrients: Protein: 6g | Carbs: 15g | Fats: 8g

Dinner: Beef Stir-Fry with Broccoli, Bell Peppers, and Brown Rice

- Ingredients: 150g beef, 1 cup broccoli, 1 bell pepper, 1 cup cooked brown rice
- Macronutrients: Protein: 30g | Carbs: 40g | Fats: 12g

Total Daily Macronutrients: Protein: 81g | Carbs: 95g | Fats: 47g | Calories: 1127

Day 5

Breakfast: Greek Yogurt with Granola and Mixed Berries

- Ingredients: 1 cup Greek yogurt, 1/2 cup granola, 1/2 cup mixed berries
- Macronutrients: Protein: 20g | Carbs: 40g | Fats: 7g

Lunch: Chicken Caesar Salad with Whole Grain Croutons

- Ingredients: 100g grilled chicken breast, Romaine lettuce, Parmesan cheese, whole grain croutons, Caesar dressing
- Macronutrients: Protein: 30g | Carbs: 20g | Fats: 15g

Snack: Mixed Nuts and Dried Fruit

- Ingredients: 1/4 cup mixed nuts, 1/4 cup dried fruit
- Macronutrients: Protein: 5g | Carbs: 20g | Fats: 15g

Dinner: Baked Cod, Sweet Potato, and Green Beans

- Ingredients: 150g cod fillet, 1 medium sweet potato, 1 cup green beans
- Macronutrients: Protein: 28g | Carbs: 45g | Fats: 5g

Total Daily Macronutrients: Protein: 83g | Carbs: 125g | Fats: 42g | Calories: 1210

Day 6

Breakfast: Smoothie with Spinach, Banana, Protein Powder, and Almond Milk

- Ingredients: 1 cup spinach, 1 banana, 1 scoop protein powder, 1 cup almond milk
- Macronutrients: Protein: 25g | Carbs: 30g | Fats: 4g

Lunch: Quiche with Mixed Green Salad

- Ingredients: 1 slice quiche, mixed greens, olive oil vinaigrette
- Macronutrients: Protein: 20g | Carbs: 30g | Fats: 18g

Snack: Rice Cakes with Peanut Butter and Greek yogurt

- Ingredients: 2 rice cakes, 2 tbsp peanut butter
- Macronutrients: Protein: 23g | Carbs: 34g | Fats: 10g

Dinner: Vegetarian Chili with Kidney Beans and Cornbread

- Ingredients: 1 cup vegetarian chili (kidney beans, tomatoes, onions), 1 slice cornbread
- Macronutrients: Protein: 15g | Carbs: 55g | Fats: 10g

Total Daily Macronutrients: Protein: 83g | Carbs: 149g | Fats: 44g | Calories: 1368

Day 7

Breakfast: Egg and Vegetable Omelet with Whole Grain Toast

- Ingredients: 2 eggs, mixed vegetables (bell peppers, onions, tomatoes), 1 slice whole grain toast
- Macronutrients: Protein: 20g | Carbs: 15g | Fats: 12g

Lunch: Grilled Salmon Salad with Avocado

- Ingredients: 150g grilled salmon, mixed greens, 1/2 avocado, vinaigrette dressing
- Macronutrients: Protein: 30g | Carbs: 20g | Fats: 20g

Snack: Greek Yogurt with Honey and Almonds

- Ingredients: 1 cup Greek yogurt, 1 tbsp honey, 10 almonds
- Macronutrients: Protein: 18g | Carbs: 25g | Fats: 6g

Dinner: Roast Chicken with Roasted Vegetables

- Ingredients: 150g roast chicken, carrots, onions, Brussels sprouts
- Macronutrients: Protein: 35g | Carbs: 30g | Fats: 15g

Total Daily Macronutrients: Protein: 103g | Carbs: 90g | Fats: 53g | Calories: 1249

Note: The macronutrient and calorie values are approximate and may vary based on the exact size and brand of ingredients used. It's important to tailor the portion sizes and ingredients according to individual dietary needs, preferences, and specific health conditions. You may require higher calories and protein intake based on individual needs. Talking to a registered dietician to get specifics on your caloric needs may be beneficial.

This meal plan is designed to provide a balanced diet focusing on protein for muscle maintenance, carbohydrates for energy, and healthy fats for overall health. You can adjust the quantities and ingredients to suit personal preferences and nutritional requirements. Overall, aim to vary protein sources, incorporate a wide range of vegetables and fruits, and choose whole grains for complex carbohydrates.

As you incorporate these meal planning and preparation strategies into your routine, remember that each nutritious meal, each hydrating drink, and each healthy snack is fueling your strength training efforts. It's nourishing your body, supporting your muscles, and contributing to your overall health. So, whether you're savoring a home-cooked meal, enjoying a healthy snack, or deciphering a food label, appreciate the role that each plays in your strength training routine. After all, in the symphony of strength training, nutrition plays a leading role, orchestrating a harmony of benefits for your body, your health, and your well-being.

9

CULTIVATING A STRENGTH TRAINING MINDSET: THE POWER OF POSITIVITY, GOAL-SETTING, AND CELEBRATING WINS

THE POWER OF A POSITIVE MINDSET

There's a well-known saying attributed to Henry Ford: "Whether you think you can, or you think you can't - you're right." This simple phrase encapsulates the profound impact of our mindset on our actions and outcomes. In the context of strength training, embracing a positive mindset can be as crucial as the weights you lift or the exercises you perform. It shapes your attitude toward your routine, influences your commitment, and, ultimately, determines your success.

Benefits of Optimism

Consider a sunflower. No matter where it's planted, it grows tall and sturdy, reaching for the light and radiating beauty. This is the essence of optimism - focusing on the light, the positive, even amidst challenges. Research supports this analogy, associating optimism with various health benefits.

According to a study published in the American Journal of Epidemiology, optimists tend to have healthier behaviors - they're more likely to engage in regular physical activity, maintain a healthier diet, and better manage stress. Furthermore, a positive outlook encourages resilience, helping you navigate the ups and downs of your strength training journey with grace and perseverance.

Visualization Techniques

Visualization, or mental imagery, is a powerful tool that can help cultivate a positive mindset. It's like running a rehearsal in your mind, preparing you for the actual performance. Athletes across various sports use this technique to enhance their performance, and it can be equally effective for strength training.

Start by finding a quiet, comfortable place to focus without interruptions. Close your eyes and imagine yourself performing your strength training routine. Visualize each exercise and movement. Feel the weight in your hands, the tension in your muscles, and the sweat on your brow.

But don't stop there. Imagine the satisfaction of completing your workout, the sense of accomplishment, the strength in your body. This positive reinforcement can boost your motivation, making your workout routine not just an obligation but a source of joy and fulfillment.

Positive Affirmations

Positive affirmations are like your personal cheerleaders, encouraging you and boosting your self-belief. They are positive statements that you repeat to yourself, reinforcing your ability to achieve your strength training goals.

Start by identifying any negative thoughts you may have, such as "I'm too weak" or "I'll never be able to do this." Then, reframe these thoughts into positive affirmations, such as "I am getting stronger every day" or "I can do this."

Repeat these affirmations to yourself regularly, particularly during your workouts. Write them on sticky notes and place them around your home. Make them your phone or computer wallpaper. The goal is to immerse yourself in positivity, fueling your strength training journey with self-belief and optimism.

Cultivating a positive mindset is like planting a seed in fertile soil. With the right care - optimism, visualization, and positive affirmations - this seed can grow into a sturdy tree, providing shade and fruit along your strength training journey. But remember, as with any tree, growth takes time. So, be patient with yourself, nourish your positive mindset, and trust your ability to grow, thrive, and reach for the sky.

SETTING ACHIEVABLE STRENGTH TRAINING GOALS

SMART Goal Framework

Consider a lighthouse guiding ships safely to shore. Its light is steady, reliable, and visible from a distance, providing a clear target for the sailors. In the context of strength training, setting SMART goals can provide a similar guiding light, leading you toward your fitness objectives in a structured and achievable manner.

The SMART framework is an acronym that stands for Specific, Measurable, Achievable, Relevant, and Time-bound. Each of these components contributes to forming a complete, well-defined goal.

- Specific: Instead of setting a vague goal like "I want to get stronger," a specific goal might be "I want to be able to do 10 push-ups." This clarity provides a definitive target to aim for.
- Measurable: A measurable goal is quantifiable, allowing you to track your progress. For instance, "I want to do 30 minutes of strength training three times a week." You can tick off each workout on your calendar, clearly seeing your progress.
- Achievable: An achievable goal is realistic and within your capabilities. If you're new to strength training, a goal like "I want to lift 100 pounds" might not be achievable. Instead, "I want to start with 2-pound weights and gradually increase the weight as I grow stronger" might be more suitable.
- Relevant: A relevant goal aligns with your broader life objectives. If your overall aim is to improve your health and

mobility, a relevant strength training goal could be "I want to strengthen my leg muscles to improve my balance and reduce the risk of falls."

- Time-bound: A time-bound goal has a deadline, creating a sense of urgency and motivation. For example, "I want to be able to do 10 push-ups within the next three months."

By setting SMART goals, you can navigate your strength training routine with purpose and direction, making steady progress towards your fitness aspirations.

Importance of Realistic Goals

Imagine standing at the base of a towering mountain, planning to reach the peak. It's a daunting task, but by breaking it down into smaller, achievable segments - base camp, mid-point, final ascent - the climb becomes more manageable. Similarly, setting realistic goals in your strength training routine makes the path to fitness success more achievable.

Realistic goals take into account your current fitness level, any health conditions, and your lifestyle. They push you to improve, but not to the point of strain or injury. For instance, if you haven't exercised in a while, a realistic goal might be completing two 20-minute strength training sessions weekly. As your fitness improves, you can adjust your goals, increasing the duration or frequency of your workouts.

Remember, the aim is not to compare yourself to others or to strive for perfection. It's about doing what's right for you, challenging yourself within your limits, and celebrating each step forward.

Tracking Progress

Just as a gardener keeps a record of which plants are growing, which need more care, and which are ready to bloom, tracking your progress in strength training provides valuable insights into your growth and areas that need more attention.

This can be as simple as keeping a workout log, noting down the exercises you performed, the weights you used, and the number of sets and repetitions. You can also note down how you felt during and after the workout, any difficulties you encountered, and how you overcame them.

Over time, this logbook becomes a tangible record of your progress, showcasing your improvements, the challenges you've overcome, and the milestones you've achieved. It serves as a source of motivation, reminding you of how far you've come and inspiring you to keep going.

Setting achievable goals, ensuring they're realistic, and tracking your progress are critical components of your strength training routine. They provide direction, motivation, and a sense of achievement, propelling you forward in your fitness endeavors. So, whether you're lifting weights, balancing on one leg, or stretching after a workout, remember that each movement, each effort, is a step towards achieving your goals, enriching your health, and enhancing your life.

CELEBRATING PROGRESS AND ACCOMPLISHMENTS

Reward System

Think of your favorite game. Each level completed and each challenge overcome earns you points or rewards, adding to the excitement and motivation to proceed further. Similarly, setting up a reward system for your strength training goals can boost your motivation and make your fitness routine more enjoyable.

The rewards you choose can be as simple or elaborate as you like. It could be a relaxing bath after a workout, a new book after a week of consistent workouts, or even a weekend getaway after achieving a major fitness milestone. The key is to choose rewards that are meaningful to you and that reinforce your commitment to your fitness goals.

Remember, the reward is not just about the prize at the end. It's about recognizing your efforts, celebrating your discipline, and taking a moment to acknowledge the work you're putting into your health and well-being.

Non-Scale Victories

Within health and fitness, the scale often gets the spotlight. However, non-scale victories often provide a more accurate and encouraging picture of your progress when it comes to strength training.

Non-scale victories are those triumphant moments that can't be measured by a weight scale but are equally, if not more, significant. It could be noticing an improvement in your posture, feeling more energized during the day, sleeping better at night, or easily carrying a heavy grocery bag. Each of these victories is a testament to your improving strength and health.

So, while the scale may sometimes stall, these non-scale victories provide tangible proof of your progress, reminding you of the many benefits of strength training beyond weight loss.

Reflective Journaling

In the hustle and bustle of daily life, we often forget to pause and reflect on our experiences. Reflective journaling provides an opportunity to do just that. It's equivalent to hitting the pause button on a busy day, offering you a space to express your thoughts, document your progress, and celebrate your victories.

Keeping a journal of your strength training journey allows you to track your workouts, record your feelings, and note any challenges or breakthroughs. But more importantly, it provides a medium through which you can express gratitude for your body and its capabilities, celebrate your progress, and motivate yourself to keep going.

Writing in your journal after each workout can be therapeutic, helping you unwind and process your experiences. Over time, this journal becomes a record of your strength training journey, marking each step you've taken towards improved health and strength.

Celebrating progress and accomplishments is an integral part of your strength training routine. It's about acknowledging your efforts, rejoicing in your victories, and using these positive experiences to fuel your motivation and commitment. Whether it's through setting up a reward system, celebrating non-scale victories, or journaling your experiences, each celebration adds a splash of joy to your strength training routine, painting a vibrant picture of progress, achievement, and well-being.

UNRAVELING MENTAL ROADBLOCKS TO STRENGTH TRAINING

Fear of Injury

The shadow of potential injury can loom over your strength training aspirations, acting as an intimidating roadblock. However, much like a well-designed bridge allows safe passage over a treacherous ravine, adopting safety measures in your strength training routine can help you confidently cross this roadblock.

Start by getting a thorough health check-up and discussing your strength training plans with your healthcare provider. This lays a solid foundation, ensuring your routine aligns with your health status.

Next, consider working with a certified fitness professional or physical therapist who can guide you on proper form and technique. This will ensure your movements are correct and safe, much like a skilled driving instructor ensures you adhere to road safety rules.

Finally, listen to your body. If an exercise causes pain or discomfort, it's a signal to stop and reassess. Remember, strength training is not about pushing through pain but about working within current abilities and gradually expanding them.

Perceived Lack of Time

Time, or the lack of it, can often feel like a formidable barrier to regular exercise. But let's consider time as a vast ocean. While it might seem overwhelming, dividing it into smaller portions becomes manageable.

The same principle applies to your strength training routine. Instead of trying to carve out a large chunk of time in your day, aim for shorter, more frequent sessions. Even 10 to 15 minutes of focused strength training can be beneficial, and these small pockets of time can add up significantly over a week.

To make this easier, consider incorporating strength training into your everyday activities. For instance, do a few squats while waiting for the kettle to boil, complete several standing calf raises while brushing your teeth, or perform seated leg lifts while watching your favorite television show. This way, strength training becomes a part of your daily routine rather than an additional task competing for your time.

Self-Doubt

Self-doubt can be an insidious mental barrier, subtly undermining your confidence and motivation. It's akin to a leaky faucet, slowly draining away your resolve. However, with the right mindset and strategies, you can seal this leak and bolster your self-belief.

Firstly, remember that everyone starts somewhere. You don't need to be an expert to begin strength training. With patience, persistence, and practice, you will improve over time.

Secondly, focus on your achievements, no matter how small. Each exercise you complete, each repetition you perform, is a victory to celebrate. This positive reinforcement can boost your confidence and motivate you to keep going.

Lastly, surround yourself with positivity. This could be through motivating podcasts, inspiring books, or supportive friends and family. A positive environment can significantly influence your mindset, helping you overcome self-doubt and confidently embrace your strength training routine.

Mental barriers to exercise, like fear of injury, perceived lack of time, or self-doubt, can be navigated effectively with the right approach. The strategies outlined in this chapter act like a compass, guiding you through these roadblocks and steering you toward your strength training goals.

So, as you develop your strength training routine, remember to cultivate a positive mindset, set achievable goals, celebrate your progress, and navigate mental barriers with confidence. With this approach, you're training not just your body but also your mind, creating a synergy of physical and mental strength that fuels your overall health and well-being.

As we turn the page to the next chapter, let's carry forward this holistic perspective, ready to explore how a supportive community can enhance your strength training experience, making it more enjoyable, sustainable, and rewarding.

10

THE POWER OF COMMUNITY IN STRENGTH TRAINING

I magine a flock of geese flying in a V formation, each bird benefiting from the uplift of air provided by the bird in front. This is the essence of a supportive community - individuals coming together, providing lift and momentum to each other, making the journey easier and more enjoyable. A supportive community can provide motivation, encouragement, and a sense of camaraderie, enhancing your experience and fostering long-term commitment to your strength training journey.

FINDING YOUR STRENGTH TRAINING SUPPORT NETWORK

Local Fitness Groups

Consider your local community center, park, or recreational facility. These venues often host fitness groups catering to different interests and ability levels. From group exercise classes to walking clubs, these local fitness groups offer a social platform to engage in physical activity, much like a book club, which provides a social setting for discussing literature.

Participating in a local fitness group allows you to connect with like-minded individuals, share experiences, and learn from each other. It's an opportunity to form friendships, foster accountability, and create a sense of belonging. It's akin to joining a gardening club, where you nurture plants and relationships.

Online Communities

In today's digital age, the world is at our fingertips. The internet offers a plethora of online communities centered around fitness and health. From forums and social media groups to fitness apps and online classes, these platforms provide a virtual space for individuals to connect, much like an online book club connects book lovers from around the world.

Joining an online community offers flexibility and convenience. You can participate from the comfort of your home at a time that suits you. These platforms provide a wealth of resources, from workout tips and motivational stories to expert advice and Q&A sessions. It's like having a personal fitness library, offering a wealth of knowledge and support.

Family Involvement

Don't underestimate the power of your immediate circle. Your family, whether it's your spouse, children, or grandchildren, can be an integral part of your support network. Involving them in your strength training routine is like involving them in a family project. It strengthens bonds, encourages shared experiences, and fosters mutual support.

Family members can join you in your workouts, serve as workout buddies, or provide moral support. They can celebrate your milestones and encourage you when the going gets tough. It's akin to cooking a meal together, where each person plays a part, contributing to a nourishing and enjoyable outcome.

Finding your strength training support network is like assembling a jigsaw puzzle. Each piece - local fitness groups, online communities, family involvement - adds to the picture, creating a comprehensive network that supports and enriches your strength training experience. So, whether you're lifting weights, balancing on one leg, or performing a seated leg extension, remember that you're not alone. You're part of a community, a flock of geese flying in formation, each member providing lift and momentum to the others, making the journey easier, more enjoyable, and more rewarding.

TIPS FOR FAMILY AND CAREGIVERS

Encouraging Regular Exercise

Family members and caregivers play a pivotal role in encouraging seniors to incorporate regular exercise into their lifestyle. This task is like a gardener encouraging the growth of a plant by providing it with water, sunlight, and nutrients. Your role is to provide the necessary encouragement, guidance, and support to facilitate the growth of a regular exercise routine.

To do this, it's important to highlight the value of strength training and its impact on overall health and well-being. Emphasize the benefits such as increased mobility, improved balance, enhanced energy levels, and boosted mood. It's like pointing out a blossoming flower's beauty, highlighting the positive outcome of regular care.

Additionally, caregivers can actively participate in the exercise routine, creating fun and camaraderie. This shared experience can make exercise sessions more enjoyable and something to look forward to. Consider it like a shared gardening session, where gardening becomes a pleasant activity rather than a chore.

Safety Precautions

While encouraging regular exercise, it's equally important to ensure that safety precautions are in place. This responsibility is similar to that of a lifeguard watching over swimmers, ensuring everyone's safety while they enjoy their swim.

Firstly, it's crucial to ensure that the exercise area is safe. This means having a clear and open space, free from clutter that could cause trips and falls. It's like clearing a pathway in a garden, removing any obstacles that could hinder the growth of plants.

Secondly, ensure that any equipment used is in good condition, safe, and appropriate for the senior's fitness level. This could include weights, resistance bands, or a sturdy chair for balance exercises. It's akin to providing the right gardening tools and facilitating the gardening process.

Lastly, caregivers should be aware of the senior's medical history and any specific health concerns. This information is essential in tailoring the exercise routine to meet the individual's needs and capabilities. It's much like understanding a plant's specific needs, ensuring it receives the right amount of sunlight, water, and nutrients for optimal growth.

Emotional Support

Emotional support is another crucial aspect of family members' and caregivers' roles. It's like the sun's warmth, providing comfort and encouragement for the plant to grow.

Acknowledge the effort it takes for seniors to exercise regularly, especially if they're new to strength training. Express your pride in their commitment and celebrate their accomplishments, no matter how small they may seem. This validation can boost their motivation and self-confidence. It's like praising the growth of a plant, acknowledging the progress it's made.

Be there to listen to their concerns, challenges, or fears. Offering a listening ear and empathetic responses can provide immense emotional support. It's akin to providing shade for a plant on a scorching day, offering comfort and protection.

As a family member or caregiver, your role in encouraging regular exercise, ensuring safety precautions, and providing emotional support is pivotal in a senior's strength training routine. Like a gardener tending to a plant, your care and support can foster the growth of a regular exercise habit, promoting the senior's health, strength, and overall well-being.

STAYING MOTIVATED IN YOUR STRENGTH TRAINING JOURNEY

Setting New Challenges

Imagine a hiker on a trail. After reaching one peak, they're immediately drawn to the next. The sense of accomplishment from overcoming one challenge fuels the desire to take on another. Similarly, setting new challenges in your strength training routine can create a ripple of excitement and a renewed sense of purpose.

A new challenge could be anything that nudges you out of your comfort zone. It could be increasing the weight you're lifting, adding a new exercise to your routine, aiming to complete your workout in a shorter time, or committing to an additional workout session each week.

Whatever the challenge, it should be something that excites you and sparks a sense of curiosity and determination. Like the hiker standing at the foot of a new peak, ready to make the climb, you'll feel a surge of motivation each time you set a new challenge in your strength training routine.

Regularly Updating Workout Routines

Picture a river, flowing freely, constantly moving and changing its course. If the river were to stop flowing, it would become stagnant. Similarly, regularly updating your workout routine keeps your strength training flowing, preventing it from becoming stagnant or monotonous.

Updating your workout routine can take various forms. You might switch the order of your exercises or introduce new ones. You could alternate between different types of workouts - for instance, adjusting from full-body workouts to ones focused on upper-body exercises one day, followed by a lower-body workout the next. Maybe you decide to experiment with different types of equipment, like resistance bands or stability balls.

Regular updates keep your workouts interesting and challenge your muscles in new ways, enhancing the effectiveness of your strength training. Like the river that carves out new paths, you'll find yourself exploring new aspects of strength training, keeping your routine fresh and engaging.

Recognizing the Benefits

Imagine watching a seedling grow into a flourishing plant. Over time, you start to notice the buds forming and then the blossoms blooming. Recognizing these changes fills you with a sense of joy and satisfaction. Similarly, recognizing the benefits of your strength training routine can significantly enhance your motivation.

These benefits could be physical, such as increased strength, improved balance, or enhanced flexibility. You might notice changes in your body, like improved posture or increased muscle tone. You could find that your daily activities, like climbing stairs or carrying groceries, become easier.

The benefits could also be mental or emotional. Perhaps you notice an uplift in your mood after your workouts, or maybe you find that you're sleeping better. You could experience a boost in self-confidence as you overcome challenges and reach new milestones.

Recognizing these benefits is like pausing to admire the blossoming plant. It's a moment to appreciate the fruits of your labor and to see the tangible results of your efforts. Each benefit you recognize serves as a reminder of why you started strength training in the first place, reinforcing your commitment and fueling your motivation to continue.

Motivation can be as vital as the weights you lift or the exercises you perform. Whether setting new challenges, updating your workout routine, or recognizing the benefits, each strategy plays a key role in fueling your motivation. So, as you take on new challenges, explore different exercises, and witness the fruits of your labor, remember that each step and each achievement is a testament to your strength, commitment, and incredible journey toward health and vitality.

SHARING YOUR STRENGTH TRAINING SUCCESS STORIES

Social Media Sharing

Imagine a digital stage, accessible to people worldwide, where you can showcase your fitness journey. Social media platforms like Facebook, Instagram, and Twitter offer such a stage. Sharing your strength training success stories on social media documents your progress and motivates and inspires others.

Think of your first successful push-up or the day you reached a personal best in your dumbbell lift. These victories, big or small, are moments of celebration that deserve to be shared. A simple post, a photo, or a short video can capture these achievements, creating a digital scrapbook of your strength training milestones.

Sharing your stories on social media also opens up avenues for support and encouragement. Likes, shares, comments, and messages from friends, family, and even strangers can boost your motivation and reinforce your commitment. In essence, social media can act as a global fitness community, bringing people together, fostering a sense of camaraderie, and promoting a culture of health and fitness.

Testimonials in Local Groups

Let's shift the focus from the digital stage to the local arena. Local fitness groups, community centers, and senior clubs often provide opportunities for members to share their experiences. Contributing your strength training success stories to these local groups can have a significant impact.

Consider the power of a face-to-face conversation and the intimacy of sharing experiences in person. Your stories can inspire others in your community, showing them the tangible benefits of strength training. Whether it's an improvement in balance, an increase in strength, or a boost in energy levels, your testimonials provide real-life evidence of the positive impact of strength training.

Moreover, sharing your stories in local groups can enhance your sense of belonging. It's an opportunity to connect with others, exchange tips and advice, and contribute to the group's collective knowledge. It's like adding a unique thread to a community tapestry, enriching its texture and enhancing its value.

Inspiring Others

Lastly, let's reflect on the ripple effect of your strength training success stories. By sharing your experiences, you're not just documenting your progress but also inspiring others, showing them what's possible. It's like tossing a pebble into a pond. The ripples spread out, reaching far beyond the point of impact.

Your strength training journey can inspire others to start their own, particularly those who may feel hesitant or unsure. Your stories can show them that age is not a barrier to fitness, that it's never too late to start, and that every step counts, no matter how small. Your victories can motivate them, your challenges can guide them, and your perseverance can inspire them.

By sharing your strength training success stories, you're not just celebrating your achievements but also contributing to a larger narrative of health, fitness, and vitality among seniors. It's about being a part of something bigger, making a difference, and leaving a positive mark. So, keep sharing, inspiring, and making waves in the vast pond of strength training for seniors.

Sharing your strength training success stories, whether it's through social media, local groups, or inspiring others, is a powerful way to document your progress, celebrate your victories, and contribute to the larger fitness narrative. It's about using your voice to inspire, motivate, and guide others on their strength training path. But beyond that, it's about finding connection, fostering a sense of community, and relishing the joy of shared experiences and collective growth. As we move forward, let's continue to embrace the power of sharing, the strength of community, and the joy of mutual growth.

11

EMBRACING TECHNOLOGY IN STRENGTH TRAINING

J ust as the gentle hum of a GPS guides you smoothly down the road, technology can guide us seamlessly through our fitness routines. In our modern world, technology permeates nearly every aspect of our lives. It's only fitting, then, that it should also be an ally in our pursuit of health and fitness. Let's explore how digital tools and apps can enrich your strength training routine, making it more interactive, organized, and effective.

STRENGTH TRAINING APPS AND DIGITAL TOOLS

Technology has revolutionized how we approach fitness, offering many digital tools designed to make our routines more streamlined, personalized, and engaging. These tools serve as handy companions on your strength training path, much like a Swiss Army knife, versatile and ready to assist in various situations.

Fitness Tracker Apps

Fitness tracker apps are like digital notebooks, keeping a meticulous record of your workouts, steps, calories burned, and even sleep patterns. They are a tool to measure progress, set goals, and gain insights about your health and fitness.

Apps such as MyFitnessPal, Fitbod, and JEFIT offer features tailored for strength training, including workout logs, exercise libraries, and customizable workout plans. With the added convenience of having these tools right on your smartphone or tablet, tracking your workouts becomes as easy as a few taps on a screen.

In addition, multiple brands of smart watches can help you track your activity level, workouts, heart rate, and even sleep.

Online Personal Training Platforms

Online personal training platforms bridge the gap between independent workouts and one-on-one training sessions. It's akin to having a personal trainer in your pocket, ready to guide you at your convenience.

Platforms like Trainiac, Future, and TrainHeroic connect you with certified personal trainers who develop customized workout plans based on your fitness level, goals, and preferences. These platforms often include features like video demonstrations, progress tracking, and direct messaging with your trainer. This personalized guidance can provide the motivation and accountability of a personal trainer with the flexibility of an at-home workout.

Virtual Reality Fitness

Virtual reality (VR) fitness is the frontier of fitness technology, combining immersive virtual environments with interactive workouts. It's like stepping into a fitness-themed video game, transforming your workout routine into an engaging and enjoyable experience.

VR fitness platforms like Supernatural, FitXR, and VZfit offer a variety of workout experiences, including strength training. Wearing a VR headset, you can perform workouts in stunning virtual landscapes guided by virtual coaches. It's an innovative way to make fitness fun, helping you stay motivated and enjoy your strength training routine.

Fitness tracker apps, online personal training platforms, and virtual reality fitness are digital tools that can elevate your strength training routine. They provide a blend of convenience, personalization, and engagement that can make your fitness journey more enjoyable and effective.

ONLINE STRENGTH TRAINING RESOURCES

YouTube Fitness Channels

Let's first turn our attention to a platform that has become synonymous with online video content - YouTube. YouTube fitness channels can serve as a virtual fitness library, readily available and easily accessible. With a diverse array of fitness channels, YouTube caters to a multitude of fitness levels, workout styles, and personal preferences.

Channels such as HASFit, FitnessBlender, Bob and Brad, and Senior Fitness with Meredith offer strength training workouts and tips suited for seniors. These workouts often come with clear instructions, visual demonstrations, and modifications, making them suitable for different ability levels. The option to pause, rewind, or replay the videos allows you to exercise at your own pace, ensuring comprehension and safety.

Thus, YouTube fitness channels offer an interactive and flexible platform to guide your strength training routine, much like a fitness DVD, but with the added benefits of variety, accessibility, and user-friendly features.

Online Fitness Blogs

If you're more inclined towards reading, online fitness blogs can be an invaluable resource. These blogs often bring together expert advice, workout ideas, motivational stories, and practical tips, much like an online fitness magazine tailored to your interests.

Blogs such as Senior Fitness, Nia Shanks, and Strength Training for Seniors offer a wealth of information on strength training, from the basic principles and techniques to more advanced topics. Whether you're looking for advice on starting strength training, tips for injury prevention, or ideas for overcoming plateaus, these blogs have you covered.

In addition, many of these blogs offer the opportunity to join a mailing list, delivering the latest posts directly to your inbox. This means you can stay updated with new content and information, ensuring steady inspiration and guidance for your strength training routine.

Webinars and Online Courses

Webinars and online courses take fitness education to a new level, offering structured learning experiences from the comfort of your home. Think of them as a virtual fitness classroom where you can deepen your understanding of strength training and enhance your skills.

Platforms such as Coursera, Udemy, and FutureLearn offer online courses on topics ranging from exercise physiology to fitness nutrition. These courses often include video lectures, reading materials, quizzes, and peer discussion forums, providing a comprehensive learning experience.

Webinars, on the other hand, offer live, interactive sessions with fitness experts. They often include a presentation followed by a Q&A session, giving you the opportunity to have your questions answered in real time.

Whether it's a webinar or an online course, these platforms offer a structured, in-depth learning experience. They allow you to delve deeper into the world of strength training, equipping you with knowledge and skills to enhance your fitness routine.

YouTube fitness channels, online fitness blogs, webinars, and online courses offer a plethora of resources to support your strength training routine. They provide a blend of visual content, written information, and structured learning experiences, catering to different learning styles and preferences. With these resources at your fingertips, you can confidently navigate your strength training routine, equipped with the knowledge, inspiration, and guidance to reach your fitness goals.

HOW TECHNOLOGY CAN ENHANCE YOUR STRENGTH TRAINING

Progress Tracking

In the grand theater of fitness, progress tracking is the spotlight, shining a light on your achievements and illuminating the path forward. Modern technology offers intuitive digital tools, making progress tracking not just a routine task but a dynamic and motivating part of your strength training regimen.

Fitness apps and wearable devices provide detailed analytics of your workouts, recording data like the amount of weight lifted, repetitions performed, and rest periods taken. This data serves as a digital mirror, reflecting your performance and revealing patterns that may otherwise go unnoticed.

For instance, you might notice that your energy levels peak in the mornings, making it an optimal time for your strength training sessions. Or you may find that you can perform more repetitions of an exercise after a restful night's sleep. These insights enable you to tailor your routine to your unique needs and rhythms, enhancing its effectiveness.

Moreover, progress tracking provides tangible evidence of your achievements. Seeing your weights increase over time or your repetitions grow in number is a testament to your efforts. These visible signs of progress serve as motivators, fueling your determination and boosting your self-belief.

Virtual Coaching

Picture a world where professional guidance is available at the click of a button. Virtual coaching makes this a reality, bringing expert advice and personalized programs into your living room. It's like having a personal strength training coach who's available at your convenience, providing instruction, feedback, and motivation.

Through online platforms or fitness apps, virtual coaches can guide you through workouts, demonstrate correct form, and provide real-time feedback. These expert insights can help you avoid common pitfalls and maximize the benefits of your strength training exercises.

Additionally, virtual coaching offers a personalized approach. Your coach can design a strength training program that aligns with your fitness level, health conditions, and personal goals. They can also adapt the program as you progress, ensuring it remains challenging and effective.

Another benefit is that virtual coaching provides accountability. Regular check-ins and progress reviews with your coach can keep you motivated and committed to your strength training routine. It's like having a workout buddy who not only cheers you on but also provides expert advice and constructive feedback.

Access to Diverse Workouts

Imagine a library where, instead of books, the shelves are filled with diverse workout routines. Technology provides such a library, offering a wealth of strength training routines at your fingertips. With access to such a diverse range of workouts, your strength training routine can remain fresh, engaging, and challenging.

Online platforms, fitness apps, and social media channels offer many workout ideas. The options are vast and varied, from bodyweight exercises to resistance band workouts, from balance exercises to flexibility routines.

This diversity allows you to experiment with different exercises, keeping your routine exciting and preventing workout boredom. It also ensures that your muscles are challenged in different ways, contributing to a well-rounded fitness regimen.

Having access to diverse workouts allows you to adapt your routine to your circumstances. If you're traveling, for instance, you can opt for bodyweight exercises that require no equipment. Or, if you're recovering from an injury, you can choose low-impact exercises that are gentle on your body.

Technology can significantly enhance your strength training routine. Through progress tracking, you can gain insights into your performance and celebrate your achievements. Virtual coaching provides expert guidance, personalized programs, and accountability. Access to diverse workouts keeps your routine fresh and adaptable. Together, these benefits can make your strength training routine effective, enjoyable, motivating, and uniquely suited to you.

SAFETY MEASURES WHEN USING FITNESS TECHNOLOGY

Protecting Personal Data

In our digitally interconnected world, the safeguarding of personal data is of utmost importance. Like a lock securing your home, robust safety measures protect your personal information from unauthorized access.

Fitness technology platforms often require you to share personal data, including health metrics, workout statistics, and, in some cases, even location data. Therefore, it's crucial to ensure that these platforms use reliable security measures to protect this sensitive information.

Before signing up for any fitness app or online platform, thoroughly review its privacy policies. Though often filled with legal jargon, these documents reveal how your data will be collected, used, and protected. Look for platforms that use encryption, a method that scrambles your data to prevent unauthorized access.

Also, be mindful of the data you share. While providing certain information for personalized workouts may be necessary, avoid sharing unnecessary personal details. It's like giving out your house keys; you wouldn't hand them to just anyone.

Ensuring Physical Safety

While technology brings fitness training into the comfort of your home, ensuring that your environment is safe for workouts is essential. Consider it like setting up a mini gym in your living room, where safety and convenience go hand in hand.

Ensure that your workout space is clear, open, and free from clutter that might cause trips or falls. If you're using fitness equipment like weights or resistance bands, store them safely after use to avoid accidents.

Also, remember that while virtual coaches can guide you through exercises, they can't always correct your form or spot potential risks. Therefore, it's crucial to listen to your body. If an exercise causes discomfort or feels too challenging, it's okay to modify it or take a break.

Avoiding Over-reliance on Tech Tools

While fitness technology can enhance your strength training routine, it's important not to become overly dependent on it. Consider it like using a map for navigation; while the map is helpful, it's also important to look up and take in the surroundings.

For instance, while fitness trackers provide valuable data about your workouts, they should not replace your body's feedback. No device knows your body better than you do. If you're feeling exhausted, take a rest day, even if your fitness tracker shows you haven't met your daily goal.

Similarly, while virtual coaching can provide expert guidance, it's not a substitute for healthcare advice. Always consult with a healthcare provider before starting any new fitness program.

Fitness technology is a tool, not a master. It's there to assist you, not control you. Use it to enhance your strength training routine while also listening to your body and making informed decisions about your health.

With the explosion of digital tools and resources, fitness technology has transformed the landscape of strength training, making it more accessible, personalized, and interactive. Whether it's tracking your progress with a fitness app, getting personalized coaching online, or exploring diverse workouts through virtual reality, technology offers numerous ways to enhance your strength training routine.

However, as we embrace the digital age in our fitness journey, it's important to navigate this terrain safely. This involves protecting our personal data, ensuring our physical safety during workouts, and not becoming overly reliant on tech tools. With these safety measures in place, we can leverage the power of technology to enrich our strength training routine, all while ensuring our safety and well-being.

As we turn to the next chapter, we'll continue to explore the multifaceted world of strength training for seniors, delving into the often-overlooked but equally important aspects of flexibility and balance. After all, strength training is not just about building muscle power; it's also about creating a harmonious balance of strength, flexibility, and stability. So, let's continue to learn, grow, and strengthen ourselves, one step, one rep, one breath at a time.

12

THE ROLE OF FLEXIBILITY, MOBILITY, AND BALANCE

I magine being a skilled gymnast, displaying an impressive range of motion, and performing intricate routines with grace and fluidity. Now, while we may not all aspire to be gymnasts, their dedication to flexibility is something we can all benefit from, especially as we age. Flexibility, or the ability of a muscle to move through a specific range of motion, and mobility, which is the range of motion around our joints, plays a surprisingly significant role in our daily activities and overall quality of life. In this chapter, we will explore the importance of flexibility and mobility, its impact on posture, and its connection to injury prevention.

If you haven't yet, make sure to get your free copy of "5 Essential Daily Exercises for Posture," which is available at the beginning of this book!

UNDERSTANDING FLEXIBILITY AND ITS IMPORTANCE

Role in Daily Activities

Think about your daily routine. It may involve bending to tie your shoelaces, reaching up to a high shelf to retrieve a book, or twisting to look over your shoulder while reversing your car. Each of these actions requires a certain degree of flexibility and mobility.

These fitness components enhance your ability to perform strength training exercises correctly. They allow you to maintain the correct posture, achieve the full range of movement, and thereby maximize the effectiveness of each exercise. For instance, having good flexibility in your hamstrings and hips allows you to perform a deadlift movement with proper form, engaging the right muscles and helping avoid injury.

Impact on Posture

Imagine a puppet held upright by a network of tightly pulled strings. Now, visualize what happens if one of those strings loses its tension. The puppet's posture would sag on one side. Our muscles work similarly, maintaining our body's posture and alignment.

When muscles are stiff and tight, they can pull on our joints and lead to poor posture. For example, tight chest muscles can pull your shoulders forward, causing a hunched posture. On the other hand, improved flexibility allows for better muscular balance and alignment, contributing to improved posture.

Maintaining good posture is not just about looking confident. It also reduces strain on our muscles and joints, enhances lung capacity, and improves circulation. Therefore, by improving flexibility, you can enhance your posture and reap these associated benefits.

Connection to Injury Prevention

Imagine walking on a slippery surface. Suddenly, your foot slides forward. If your leg muscles are adequately flexible, they can stretch to accommodate this unexpected movement. However, if they are excessively tight, the sudden pull might exceed their stretch capacity, leading to a muscle strain or tear.

This example illustrates how flexibility can contribute to injury prevention. Flexible muscles are less likely to be injured as they can absorb the impact of sudden movements or falls. This is particularly important for seniors, as flexibility tends to decrease with age, and injuries can take longer to heal.

Moreover, flexibility can play a crucial role in helping to prevent overuse injuries in strength training. As you perform repetitive movements in strength training exercises, muscles can become tight and imbalanced. This may pull your joints out of optimal alignment. Regular flexibility training can help maintain balanced muscle tension around joints, reducing the risk of these overuse injuries.

Flexibility plays a pivotal role in our daily activities, posture, and injury prevention. Incorporating flexibility training into your routine can enhance your strength training performance, maintain good posture, and potentially help reduce the risk of injuries.

FLEXIBILITY EXERCISES FOR SENIORS

Gentle Yoga Poses

Yoga, a practice steeped in ancient wisdom, intertwines the body and mind, promoting flexibility and tranquility. For seniors embarking on a strength training regimen, incorporating gentle yoga poses can enhance flexibility, making it a valuable addition to their fitness routine.

Consider the Tree Pose, which cultivates balance while stretching the thighs, torso, and shoulders. Or the Cat-Cow Pose, a gentle flow that enhances spinal flexibility. The Warrior Pose, in its various forms, stretches the hips, chest, and shoulders while also strengthening the legs.

These poses, among others, can be modified to accommodate varying fitness levels and mobility ranges. Using props like yoga blocks, straps, or a sturdy chair can make these poses accessible and safe for seniors.

Remember, the goal isn't to contort your body into complex poses but to gently stretch your muscles, enhancing their flexibility. Listen to your body, move within your comfort zone, and allow yoga practice to unfold a world of greater flexibility and serenity in your strength training routine.

Pilates Movements

Pilates, a system of exercises designed to improve physical strength and flexibility, provides another avenue for seniors to enhance their flexibility. Joseph Pilates, the creator of this practice, emphasized the importance of controlled, precise movements, and this principle lends itself well to the goal of enhancing flexibility.

Specific Pilates movements, such as the Spine Stretch, the Saw, and the Mermaid, focus on stretching various muscle groups. These movements require and promote flexibility in the spine, hips, and shoulders, areas vital for many daily activities and strength training exercises.

These exercises can be performed on a mat or using Pilates equipment like the Reformer. However, for seniors starting, mat exercises are recommended. They can be easily adapted to individual fitness levels and require no special equipment.

While performing these movements, the emphasis should be on control and precision rather than speed or intensity. This approach ensures that the exercises are safe and effective, maximizing the benefits of flexibility.

Stretching Techniques

Stretching is a fundamental aspect of flexibility training. It involves gently elongating muscles to increase their flexibility and range of motion. Various techniques of stretching exist, each with its unique benefits.

Static stretching involves holding a stretch for a certain period, typically 15-60 seconds. This type of stretching is beneficial after a workout, helping to cool down the body and enhance muscle flexibility. An example of a static stretch is the hamstring stretch, where you sit with one leg extended and reach towards your toes.

Dynamic stretching, on the other hand, involves moving parts of your body and gradually increasing the range of motion or speed of movement. It is ideal as a part of a warm-up routine before strength training, preparing the muscles for the workout. Leg swings, arm circles, and torso twists are examples of dynamic stretches.

Then, there is Proprioceptive Neuromuscular Facilitation (PNF), a more advanced form of stretching that involves both stretching and contracting the muscle group being targeted. While PNF is effective for increasing flexibility, it is recommended to practice it under the guidance of a trained professional, such as a physical therapist, to avoid injury and ensure correct utilization.

Incorporating these stretching techniques into your routine can significantly enhance your flexibility. Remember, flexibility is not achieved overnight but through consistent practice. Be patient with yourself, celebrate your progress, and let the journey to enhanced flexibility unfold at its own pace.

BALANCE TRAINING AND FALL PREVENTION

As we age, maintaining balance can sometimes be a tightrope walk. However, adding specific balance training exercises to your strength training routine can significantly improve stability and reduce the risk of falls. In this section, we'll explore several effective balance training exercises, including Tai Chi practices, stability ball exercises, and single-leg stands.

Tai Chi Practices

Tai Chi, an ancient Chinese martial art, has been recognized for its profound benefits in improving balance and preventing falls among seniors. Imagine a tranquil lake with gentle, steady waves caressing its surface. Practicing Tai Chi is like creating these peaceful waves within your body, with each movement flowing smoothly into the next, improving balance and coordination.

The beauty of Tai Chi lies in its simplicity and adaptability. Regardless of your fitness level, you can enjoy and benefit from Tai Chi.

Movements are slow and gentle and can be adapted to match your comfort level. Moreover, Tai Chi involves weight shifting and controlled breathing, which further aids in improving balance.

A typical Tai Chi session might include movements like 'Wave Hands like Clouds,' where you shift your weight from one leg to another in a controlled manner, or 'Grasp the Sparrow's Tail,' which involves a series of coordinated movements that gently challenge your balance. Regularly practicing these movements can significantly enhance your balance, coordination, and overall stability.

Stability Ball Exercises

Incorporating stability ball exercises into your routine is like adding a hint of spice to a recipe. It introduces an element of instability that challenges your balance, thereby strengthening the muscles that help maintain stability.

A stability ball, also known as an exercise ball, physio ball, or yoga ball, is a large, inflatable ball you can use for various exercises. When you sit or lie on the ball, your body engages several muscles to maintain balance. This strengthens these muscles and improves your overall sense of balance.

Simple stability ball exercises, such as 'Ball Marches,' where you sit on the ball and slowly march in place, or 'Ball Walks,' where you start by sitting on the ball and gradually walk your feet forward, can effectively enhance balance and stability.

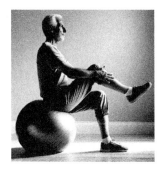

Single-Leg Stands

Standing on one leg may seem simple, but it's a powerful balance exercise. Single-leg stands strengthen the lower body, particularly the ankles and hips, which are crucial for maintaining balance.

To perform a single-leg stand:

1. Start by standing close to a wall or a sturdy chair. This will provide support if you lose balance.
2. Slowly lift one foot off the ground, maintaining balance on the other foot.
3. Aim to hold this position for about 10 seconds, then switch to the other leg. As your balance improves, you can gradually increase the duration of the stand and rely less on the support.

Balance training is a vital component of a comprehensive strength training routine for seniors. Incorporating Tai Chi practices, stability ball exercises, and single-leg stands into your routine can significantly improve balance, enhance stability, and reduce the risk of falls. So, as you continue your strength training routine, remember to balance it out with these exercises, creating a well-rounded fitness routine that promotes strength, flexibility, and stability.

INCORPORATING FLEXIBILITY AND BALANCE INTO YOUR ROUTINE

Warm-Up and Cool-Down Routines

Beginning strength training workouts with a warm-up routine helps prepare our bodies for the workout ahead. Warm-ups are not just about raising your body temperature or increasing your heart rate; they're also the perfect opportunity to improve your flexibility. Incorporating dynamic stretches, such as arm circles, leg swings, or torso twists, into your warm-up routine can gradually increase your range of motion, enhancing flexibility over time.

Now, visualize a runner crossing the finish line. They don't abruptly stop but instead gradually slow down, allowing their body to recover from the exertion of the race. This mirrors the essence of a cool-down routine following a strength training workout.

Cool-downs are not merely a period to catch your breath but also an additional opportunity to enhance flexibility. Incorporating static stretches, where you hold a stretch for 15 to 60 seconds, into your cool-down routine can help elongate your muscles, enhance flexibility, and aid in muscle recovery.

Weekly Balance Training Sessions

Imagine a gardener tending to a garden. They don't water the plants just once and forget about them; rather, they follow a regular watering schedule to ensure the plants grow and thrive. Similarly, to see significant improvements in balance, it's necessary to incorporate balance training into your weekly exercise schedule.

Designating specific days of the week for balance training can be an effective approach. This could involve practicing Tai Chi, performing stability ball exercises, or doing single-leg stands. Consistency is key in balance training. Just as a plant requires regular watering to grow, your balance skills need regular practice to improve.

Daily Stretching Habits

Finally, imagine brushing your teeth. This is a task you perform daily as part of your routine. It doesn't take long, yet it plays a crucial role in maintaining dental health. Similarly, developing daily stretching habits can play a vital role in maintaining your flexibility.

You don't need to dedicate a lot of time to stretching each day. Even a few minutes can make a difference. Take a few moments in the morning to stretch your arms and legs, or do a couple of neck and shoulder stretches during your work breaks. Before going to bed, you could do a few gentle stretches to relax your muscles and promote restful sleep.

Incorporating stretching into your daily routine ensures that it becomes a habit, not an afterthought. It's like sprinkling a bit of spice into a dish - a small amount can make a big difference. Similarly, a few minutes of daily stretching can significantly enhance your flexibility over time.

Incorporating flexibility and balance into your strength training routine is like weaving different threads into a fabric. Each thread - the warm-up and cool-down routines, the weekly balance training sessions, and the daily stretching habits - adds to the strength, flexibility, and vibrancy of the fabric. This comprehensive approach ensures that your strength training routine not only builds muscle power but also enhances flexibility, improves balance, and contributes to your overall health and well-being.

As we turn into the next chapter, let's remember that strength training is not a one-dimensional pursuit. It's a dynamic, multifaceted discipline that involves not only lifting weights but also stretching muscles, balancing on one leg, and standing tall with good posture. As we continue to explore the fascinating world of strength training, let's celebrate our progress and look forward to new discoveries, one stretch, one balance exercise, one workout at a time.

13

LONG-TERM STRENGTH TRAINING SUCCESS: TRACKING, ADJUSTING, COMMITTING, AND LIVING

Have you ever watched a sculptor at work? They start with a block of stone, seemingly unremarkable in its uniformity. Yet, with every calculated stroke, they chip away at the block, gradually revealing the masterpiece hidden within. This process of sculpting mirrors your strength training journey. You begin with an intention, and with every workout, every rep, every set, you chip away at your own block, gradually revealing the stronger, fitter, healthier version of yourself hidden within.

The art of sculpting is not just about the tools or the techniques. It's also about observation, adjustment, and patience. Similarly, the path to long-term strength training success involves tracking your progress, adjusting your routine over time, staying committed to your journey, and ultimately, living your best life with strength training.

TRACKING YOUR STRENGTH TRAINING PROGRESS

Just as a sculptor steps back periodically to observe their work from different angles, tracking your progress allows you to gain a broader perspective on your strength training journey. Here are some methods to track your progress effectively:

Fitness Journals

Think of keeping a fitness journal as writing a letter to your future self. It's a record of your workouts, triumphs, struggles, and thoughts. It's a dialogue between you and your fitness journey, offering insights to guide your actions.

What to Include in Your Fitness Journal:

- **Workout Details:** Jot down the exercises you performed, the weights you used, the number of sets and reps, and any modifications you made.
- **Physical Responses:** Note how your body responded to the workout. Did you experience any discomfort or pain? How fatigued were you after the workout? Did you feel energized?
- **Emotional Reactions:** Record your emotional responses to the workouts. Did you feel motivated, frustrated, or triumphant? How did the workout impact your mood?
- **Progress Notes:** Every few weeks, write down your progress. Are you lifting heavier weights?

Can you do more reps or sets? Are the exercises becoming easier?

Digital Fitness Trackers

In the age of technology, a digital fitness tracker is like a personal assistant, recording and analyzing your workout data. These handy devices or apps can track various aspects of your workouts, providing valuable insights into your progress.

How to Use a Digital Fitness Tracker:

1. **Record Workouts:** Most fitness trackers allow you to log your workouts, recording the type of exercise, duration, intensity, and even the calories burned.
2. **Monitor Heart Rate:** Many fitness trackers come with heart rate monitors, providing real-time data on your heart rate during workouts.

3. **Track Progress:** Fitness trackers often include features that track your progress over time, such as changes in your workout intensity, duration, or frequency.
4. **Set Goals:** Some fitness trackers allow you to set goals, like a certain number of workouts per week or a specific weight to lift, and alert you when you achieve these goals

Periodic Strength Assessments

Periodic strength assessments are like checkpoints on a road trip. They provide an opportunity to assess your progress, identify any areas for improvement, and celebrate your achievements.

How to Conduct a Strength Assessment:

- **Choose a Benchmark:** Select a few exercises that you regularly perform in your workouts. These will serve as benchmarks to assess your strengths.
- **Record Your Performance:** Every few months, record your performance in these exercises. How many reps can you do? How much weight can you lift? How does the exercise feel compared to before?
- **Compare Results:** Compare your results with previous assessments. Have you improved in terms of reps, weight, or ease of execution?
- **Celebrate Progress:** Celebrate your progress, no matter how small. Every improvement is a testament to your dedication and hard work.

By tracking your progress through fitness journals, digital fitness trackers, and periodic strength assessments, you gain valuable insights into your journey. You can observe patterns, identify areas for improvement, measure your progress, and celebrate your achievements. These strategies serve as your compass, guiding you on your path to long-term strength training success. So, keep tracking, observing, and chipping away at your block, revealing the masterpiece of strength, health, and vitality within you.

Adjusting Your Routine Over Time

Let's picture a river. Over time, it gently carves its path through the landscape, adjusting its course in response to the terrain. Similarly, your strength training regime will need to evolve and adapt over time. This continuous refinement allows your fitness regime to remain effective, challenging, and aligned with your changing needs and goals.

Introducing New Exercises

Consider a chef in a bustling kitchen. They continually experiment with new recipes and ingredients to keep the menu exciting and appealing. In the same way, introducing new exercises to your strength training routine keeps it fresh and stimulating.

New exercises stimulate different muscle groups and present new challenges to your body. This variety helps avoid plateaus, keeps you mentally engaged, and enhances the overall effectiveness of your workout routine.

To introduce new exercises, you could explore different types of strength training equipment, such as resistance bands or medicine balls. You might also consider different exercise styles, like circuit training or strength classes. Consult with a fitness professional or take advantage of online resources to ensure that new exercises are suitable for your fitness level and are performed with the correct form.

Modifying Exercise Intensity

Think of a cyclist on a hilly terrain. They shift gears to maintain speed as the gradient changes. Similarly, adjusting the intensity of your exercise is necessary to ensure that you continue to challenge your body as your fitness level improves.

Modifying exercise intensity can involve increasing the weight you lift, adding more reps or sets, or reducing rest time between sets. However, increasing intensity gradually is crucial to avoid overexertion or injuries.

As you modify the intensity, listen closely to your body. It's normal to feel a certain level of discomfort when increasing intensity, but it should never cause pain. If an increase in intensity leads to pain or extreme fatigue, it's a signal that you may need to slow down a bit.

Adapting to Physical Changes

Imagine a sailor at sea, adjusting the sails to suit the changing winds. Your strength training routine, too, will need to evolve in response to physical changes that occur as you age.

As we age, changes in our bodies, such as decreased bone density, reduced muscle mass, and increased joint stiffness, are common. These changes require adjustments to our exercise routines to remain safe, effective, and enjoyable.

For instance, if you notice increased joint stiffness, consider incorporating more low-impact exercises or spending more time on warm-ups and cool-downs. If you're experiencing a decrease in strength, you may need to reduce the weight you're lifting or increase the rest time between sets.

Remember, these adaptations are not setbacks. They are simply part of the aging process. By adapting your routine to these changes, you're not giving in to age; instead, you're taking control of your fitness and health in a way that respects and honors your body's evolving needs.

Adjusting your strength training routine over time is not just recommended but essential. It ensures that your routine continues to challenge you, respects your body's changes, and keeps your workouts exciting and enjoyable. So, just as the river carves its path, the chef experiments with recipes, the cyclist shifts gears, and the sailor adjusts the sails, don't be afraid to adapt and refine your strength training routine. It's all part of the process of carving your path to fitness, health, and vitality.

STAYING COMMITTED TO YOUR STRENGTH TRAINING JOURNEY

Commitment is the glue that holds your routine together, ensuring consistency and continuity. Much like a gardener who tends to their plants regularly, irrespective of the weather, staying committed to your strength training routine is crucial for long-term success.

Setting Realistic Goals

First, we must understand the importance of setting realistic goals. Picture a mountain climber preparing to scale a peak. They don't aim to reach the summit in a single stride but plan their ascent in stages, setting up camps along the way. Similarly, setting realistic goals in strength training is akin to planning your ascent in stages.

As mentioned earlier in this book, realistic goals are achievable, measurable, and time-bound. They reflect your current fitness level and consider your physical capabilities and limitations. For instance, if you're new to strength training, a realistic goal might be to complete two 20-minute workouts per week. As your fitness level improves, you could increase the duration, frequency, or intensity of your workouts.

Setting realistic goals serves two purposes. Firstly, it provides clear direction for your strength training routine, acting as a roadmap guiding your efforts. Secondly, it ensures that your expectations are achievable, reducing the risk of disappointment or frustration.

Building a Support Network

Next, let's consider the value of a support network. Imagine a group of cyclists on a long-distance ride. They draft off each other, taking turns at the front to shield others from the wind. This cooperative effort makes the ride more efficient and enjoyable for everyone. In strength training, a support network serves a similar function, making your fitness ride smoother and more enjoyable.

Your support network could include family members, friends, fitness buddies, or even online fitness communities. These individuals provide encouragement, motivation, and even a bit of friendly competition. They can join you in your workouts, celebrate your achievements, and provide a listening ear when you face challenges.

Moreover, a support network can foster accountability. Just as a cyclist in a group ride wouldn't abruptly stop pedaling, knowing that others are relying on you can motivate you to stick to your strength training routine.

Celebrating Small Wins

Finally, let's illuminate the importance of celebrating small wins in your strength training routine. Visualize a photographer capturing a series of snapshots throughout the day. Each snapshot might seem insignificant on its own, but together, they create a vivid picture of the day's experiences. In your strength training routine, each small win is like a snapshot, contributing to the larger picture of your progress.

A small win could be anything from completing a workout without skipping any exercises to lifting a heavier weight than before. It could be noticing an improvement in your posture or experiencing less fatigue after a workout.

Celebrating these small wins serves multiple functions. It boosts your morale, fuels your motivation, and reinforces the positive habits you're building. It allows you to enjoy the strength training process, not just the end results.

Remember, every small achievement is a testament to your effort and dedication. It's a sign that you're making progress, becoming stronger, fitter, and healthier. So, take a moment to celebrate these victories, enjoy the fruits of your labor, and appreciate your progress.

In strength training, as in life, staying committed to your routine, setting realistic goals, building a support network, and celebrating small wins are pivotal for long-term success. As you continue to nurture your routine with regular workouts, adjust your goals to reflect your progress, lean on your support network for motivation, and rejoice in your small wins, you'll find that your strength training routine becomes an integral part of your lifestyle. This becomes not just about building muscles but about cultivating health, fostering resilience, and celebrating the joy of movement.

LIVING YOUR BEST LIFE WITH STRENGTH TRAINING

Enhanced Independence

Imagine the freedom of an eagle soaring in the sky, unrestricted and unbound. Strength training can offer a similar sense of liberation, enhancing your independence and enabling you to live life on your own terms.

As you engage in regular strength training, your muscles become stronger, and your endurance improves. This newfound strength can positively impact your daily activities. Tasks that once seemed strenuous, whether it's carrying groceries, climbing stairs, or gardening, become more manageable. You rely less on others for these tasks, experiencing a sense of empowerment and self-sufficiency.

Improved strength contributes to better balance and coordination, reducing the risk of falls. This not only boosts your confidence but also promotes mobility and independence. Just as the eagle easily navigates the expansive sky, you can also navigate your daily life with greater ease and confidence.

Improved Quality of Life

Consider a beautiful tapestry. Every thread woven in contributes to its overall beauty. Similarly, every workout, every lift, and every stretch you perform contributes to the tapestry of your life, enhancing its quality.

Strength training not only enhances your physical health but also promotes mental well-being. The accomplishment of lifting a heavier weight or completing an extra rep can boost your self-esteem. Regular workouts can help regulate mood, improve sleep, and reduce stress levels, contributing to an overall sense of well-being.

Strength training can also help manage and prevent various health conditions, including diabetes, heart disease, and osteoporosis. It can also improve posture and alleviate common aches and pains. Like adding vibrant colors to a tapestry, these health benefits add vibrant days to your life, improving its quality.

Increased Longevity

Picture a river flowing endlessly, its course stretching as far as the eye can see. Strength training can similarly improve the quality of your life, promoting longevity and enhancing the golden years.

Research indicates that regular strength training can increase life-span and reduce the risk of premature mortality. It promotes heart health, maintains healthy blood sugar levels, and improves bone density, all contributing to a longer, healthier life.

Strength training promotes overall function, ensuring that you're not just living longer but also maintaining the ability to perform everyday tasks easily. It's about adding life to your years, not just years to your life.

In conclusion, strength training is more than a form of exercise. It's a lifestyle choice with far-reaching benefits. It enhances your independence, improves the quality of your life, and promotes longevity. Every workout is a step towards a stronger, healthier, and more vibrant version of yourself.

Next, we dive into the concluding chapter of this book, where we provide a comprehensive four-week strength training plan for seniors. We tie together all the concepts, principles, and strategies discussed throughout this book, providing a step-by-step guide to kick-start your strength training journey. Let's move forward together, ready to embrace this final chapter with anticipation, enthusiasm, and confidence.

14

FOUR-WEEK STRENGTH TRAINING ROUTINES: FROM BEGINNER TO ADVANCED

P erhaps you've heard the phrase, "Rome wasn't built in a day." This saying is often used to emphasize that meaningful things take time, and it's particularly apt when considering strength training. Each workout, each lift, and each rep is a brick in the structure of your improved strength and fitness. But just as a builder needs a blueprint to construct a building, you need a well-designed routine to guide your strength training efforts. This chapter will provide a blueprint for your strength training routine tailored to different fitness levels.

Remember, these routines are not set in stone. They are starting points, adaptable to your individual needs and preferences. As you gain strength and confidence, you can adjust these routines, adding more exercises, increasing the weight, or trying new workout styles. The key is making it your own, something you enjoy and look forward to. After all, the best workout routine is the one that you can stick to consistently.

If you are new to strength training, I recommend starting with the beginner program below. You can progress to the intermediate and advanced programs as your strength and fitness improve.

At the end of this chapter, you will receive app access to your free 4-week training program! This will allow you to follow along with video instructions, take notes, and track your progress over time.

A BEGINNER'S STRENGTH TRAINING ROUTINE

- 2 days a week, 20 minutes each

Workout A: Full Body Focus

- Seated Leg Extensions (2 sets of 12 reps): Sit on a chair with your feet flat on the floor. Extend your knees to straighten your legs, then slowly bend your knees to return to the starting position. This exercise targets your quadriceps. Add ankle weights to increase the challenge.
- Wall Push-Ups (2 sets of 10-12 reps): Stand facing a wall at an arm's length distance. Place your palms against the wall at shoulder height. Bend your elbows to bring your body closer to the wall, then push back to the starting position. This exercise targets your chest, shoulders, and arms.
- Seated Resistance Band Row (2 sets of 10 reps): Sit on a chair with a resistance band looped around your feet. Hold the ends of the band, then pull your hands towards your body, squeezing your shoulder blades together. Slowly return to the starting position. This exercise strengthens your back and shoulders.
- Bridges (2 sets of 12-15 reps): Lying on your back, lift your hips up as high as possible. Then, slowly return to the floor. This exercise targets your glutes and lower back.
- Supine Leg Raise (2 sets of 10-15 reps): Lying on your back, keep one leg straight as you lift up to around 45 degrees. Keep your knee straight throughout. Repeat on the opposite leg. This exercise targets your hip flexors and quadriceps.

Cool-Down:

- Walk for 5 minutes

30-60 seconds each:

- Standing Quadriceps Stretch
- Seated Hamstring Stretch
- Doorway Chest Stretch

Workout B: Full Body & Core Focus

Warm-Up (5 minutes): Marching in place, hip circles, ankle rolls.

- Chair Squats (2 sets of 10 reps): Stand in front of a chair, then slowly lower your body as if sitting down, stopping just before touching the chair. Stand back up to complete one rep. This exercise targets your glutes, quadriceps, and hamstrings.
- Heel Raises (2 sets of 10-15 reps): Stand behind a chair for support. Slowly raise your heels off the floor, then lower them back down. This exercise strengthens your calf muscles.
- Seated Leg Lifts (2 sets of 10 reps): Sit on a chair with your back straight. Slowly lift one leg until it is straight, then lower it back down. Repeat with the other leg. This exercise targets your quadriceps and core.
- Seated Overhead Shoulder Press (2 sets of 10-12 reps): While sitting in a chair, hold dumbbells or a similar form of weight at shoulder height. Press straight up overhead, then slowly lower the weight back to shoulder height. This exercise targets your shoulders and arms.
- Standing Hip Abduction (2 sets of 15-20 reps): While standing tall, swing one leg out laterally to the side, then return to the starting position. Hold onto a secure chair or counter for support. Maintain a tall posture throughout.

Repeat on the opposite leg. This exercise targets your lateral hip muscles.

Cool-Down:

- Walk for 5 minutes

30-60 seconds each:

- Standing Calf Stretch
- Seated Piriformis Stretch
- Child's Pose

Remember, during each workout, focus on performing the exercises with control and proper form. Rest for about 1 minute between sets to allow your muscles to recover. After your workout, cool down with some gentle stretching to promote flexibility and reduce muscle stiffness.

This beginner's routine is designed to be manageable and effective, introducing you to the world of strength training in a safe and gradual manner. As you get stronger and more confident, you can progress to the intermediate routine, which we will discuss in the next section.

TAKING THE NEXT STEP: AN INTERMEDIATE STRENGTH TRAINING ROUTINE

- 3 days a week, 30 minutes each

Workout A: Full Body Strength and Balance

Warm-Up (5 minutes): Start with a brisk walk or marching in place, followed by arm swings and standing hip rotations.

- Goblet Squat (3 sets of 12-15 reps): Stand in the air while holding a dumbbell or other form of weight to your chest.

Squat down as low as you feel comfortable or are able, then return to a standing position. Adjust weight as needed. This exercise targets your quadriceps, hamstrings, and glutes.

- Incline Push-Ups (3 sets of 12-15 reps): Place your hands on a sturdy table or counter, then step back until your body is at a slight angle. Lower your body towards the surface, then push back to the starting position. This exercise targets your chest and arms
- Standing Band Upright Row (3 sets of 12 reps): Stand on a resistance band with feet shoulder-width apart. Grasp the ends of the band, then pull your hands towards your body, squeezing your shoulder blades together. Slowly return to the starting position. This exercise strengthens your back and shoulders.
- Step Ups (3 sets of 15 reps): Use a sturdy step or stair around 6-8 inches in height. Step up with your right foot, then down with your left. Repeat, then complete reps on the opposite side. You can increase the height of the step or add weight to increase intensity. This exercise targets your quadriceps and glutes.
- Bird Dog (3 sets of 10 reps): Start positioned on your hands and knee. Your hips should be placed directly over your knees and shoulders directly over your hands. Place a pillow or pad under the knees if needed for comfort. Slowly raise your left arm and right leg into the air. Hold for a few seconds, then return to the starting position. Repeat on the other side.

Cool-Down:

- Walk for 5 minutes

30-60 seconds each:

- Standing Quadriceps Stretch
- Seated Hamstring Stretch

- Doorway Chest Stretch
- Cross-body shoulder stretch

Workout B: Upper Body and Core

Warm-Up (5 minutes): Begin with a gentle jog in place, followed by shoulder shrugs and knee circles.

- Plank (2 sets of 15-30 seconds): Start in a push-up position, then lower onto your forearms. Keep your body in a straight line from head to heels. This exercise targets your entire core.
- One-Arm Overhead Shoulder Press (2 sets of 10-12 reps): Start in a standing position. Hold a dumbbell in one hand at shoulder height. Press straight overhead, extending your elbow. Slowly return to the starting position. This exercise targets your shoulders, arms, and core.
- Band Face Pull (2 sets of 15-20 reps): Start in standing. Place an elastic exercise band around a pole or door jam anchor at shoulder height. As you hold each side of the band in each hand, pull your hands towards your ears into a "field goal" position. Hold for 1-2 seconds, then slowly return to starting point. This exercise targets your shoulders and upper back muscles.
- Floor Chest Press (2 sets of 10-15 reps): Start lying on the floor. While holding dumbbells or another form of hand-held weight, press the weight straight up, then control down until elbows touch the floor. Repeat. This exercise targets your chest, shoulders, and triceps.
- Dumbbell Bicep Curl (2 sets of 10-12 reps: Start in standing. Hold dumbbells by your side with arms fully straight. Palms facing forward. Bend your elbows all the way up and lift the weight towards your shoulders. Control down to the starting position. This exercise targets your bicep and forearm muscles

Cool-Down

- Walk for 5 minutes

30-60 seconds each:

- Overhead tricep stretch
- Cross-body shoulder stretch
- Doorway Chest Stretch

Workout C: Lower Body and Balance

Warm-Up (5 minutes): Start with stepping side to side, followed by arm circles and ankle rotations.

- Walking Lunges (2 sets of 10 reps each leg): Stand tall, then take a step forward with your right foot. Lower your body until your right knee is bent at a 90-degree angle. Push off your right foot to stand up, then repeat with the left foot. This exercise targets your quadriceps, hamstrings, and glutes.
- Calf Raises (2 sets of 15 reps): Stand behind a chair for support. Lift your heels off the ground, then lower them back down. This exercise strengthens your calf muscles.
- Goblet Chair Squats (2 sets of 15 reps): Start in standing, holding a weight such as a dumbbell to your chest. Slowly squat down until your bottom touches a sturdy chair, then return to standing. This exercise targets your quadriceps and glutes.
- Single-Leg Stands (2 sets of 30-60 seconds each leg): Stand behind a chair for support. Slowly lift one foot off the ground and balance on the other foot. This exercise improves balance and lower body strength.
- Tandem Balance (2 sets of 30-60 seconds each leg): Stand with one foot in front of the other so they are placed heel to toe. Balance as best you can. Increase difficulty by crossing

your arms or even more by closing your eyes. Modify by slightly holding onto a chair, wall, or counter.

Cool-Down:

- Walk for 5 minutes

30-60 seconds each:

- Child's Pose
- Overhead tricep stretch
- Doorway Chest Stretch

As you progress through this intermediate routine, focus on performing each exercise with control and proper form. Rest for about one minute between sets to allow your muscles to recover. After your workout, cool down with some gentle stretching to promote flexibility and reduce muscle stiffness. This routine is designed to challenge you more than the beginner routine, introducing new exercises and adding balance challenges. As you get stronger and more confident, you can progress to the advanced routine, which we will discuss in the next section.

LEVELING UP: AN ADVANCED STRENGTH TRAINING ROUTINE

- 4 days a week, 30-40 minutes each

Imagine standing atop a mountain peak, looking out at the breathtaking vista. The climb was challenging, but you made it. You feel stronger and more capable than ever before. This is the feeling of transitioning to an advanced strength training routine. It's an achievement, a testament to your dedication and perseverance. Now, let's explore what this advanced routine entails.

Workout A: Explosive Power and Strength: Full Body

Warm-Up (5 minutes): Begin with a brisk jog in place, a fast walk, or elliptical, followed by dynamic stretches such as leg swings and arm circles.

- Explosive Chair Squats (3 sets of 6 reps): Stand with your feet hip-width apart. Lower your body into a squat, tap your bottom to a chair, then explode upwards, standing up as fast as you can. This exercise targets your quadriceps, glutes, hamstrings, and calves while also challenging your explosive power.
- Push-Up with Shoulder Tap (3 sets of 10 reps): Start in a high plank position. Lower your body towards the floor, keeping your elbows close to your body. Push back up, then tap your left shoulder with your right hand. Repeat the push-up, then tap your right shoulder with your left hand. This exercise strengthens your chest, arms, and core while improving balance and coordination. If modification is needed, perform wall push-ups or modified push-ups with shoulder taps.
- Bent-Over Rows with Dumbbells (3 sets of 12-15 reps): Stand with a dumbbell in each hand, palms facing your torso. Bend your knees slightly and bring your torso forward by bending at the waist. Keep your back straight. Lift the dumbbells towards your body, keeping your elbows close to your body. Lower the dumbbells to the starting position. This exercise targets your back, shoulders, and arms.
- Medicine Ball Slam (3 sets of 8 reps): Start standing, with feet placed in a squat stance position or slightly wider. Have a medicine ball on the ground between your feet. Start with around 6 to 8 pounds. Squat down and pick up the medicine ball, then raise overhead and explosively throw it down to the floor. Pick up and repeat. This exercise targets your legs, arms, core, and explosive power.
- Push-Press (3 sets of 6 reps): Start in a standing position, with feet in a squat stance position. Hold a pair of dumbbells at shoulder height. Perform a mini-squat, then quickly stand

up. Simultaneously press the dumbbells overhead, using the momentum gained from standing up. Control the dumbbells back to shoulder height, then repeat. This exercise targets your quads, shoulders, and explosive power.

Cool-Down:

- Walk for 5 minutes

30-60 seconds each:

- Standing Quadriceps Stretch
- Seated Hamstring Stretch
- Doorway Chest Stretch
- Seated Piriformis Stretch

Workout B: Core Stability and Flexibility

Warm-Up (5 minutes): Start with a fast walk or jog in place, followed by dynamic stretches such as torso twists and hip circles.

- Plank with Leg Lift (3 sets of 10 reps each leg): Start in a high plank position. Keeping your core engaged, lift your right leg off the ground. Lower it back down, then repeat with your left leg. This exercise targets your entire core and challenges your stability. To modify, perform with your hands on a bench or wall.
- Dead Bug (3 sets of 10 reps each leg): Start lying on your back, with your arms straight up in the air and your knees up in the air so that they are directly over your hips. Knees and hips should be bent to 90 degrees. Simultaneously lift your right arm overhead and extend your left leg out. Keep your core brace and lower back firmly against the floor. Return to the starting position, then repeat on the other side. This exercise targets your core and coordination.
- Bird Dog (3 sets of 10 reps each side): Start in a tabletop position, with your hands under your shoulders and your

knees under your hips. Extend your right arm and left leg simultaneously, keeping your body balanced. Return to the starting position, then repeat with your left arm and right leg. This exercise targets your core and improves balance.

- Suitcase Carry (3 sets of 30 seconds on each side): Hold a heavy weight in one hand by your side (e.g., a dumbbell, milk jug, etc.). Stand upright with a tall posture and engaged core. Steadily walk straight, then turn around using the opposite hand. This exercise challenges your core, grip strength, and stability.
- Seated Hamstring Stretch (2 sets of 60 seconds each leg): Sit on the ground with one leg extended and the other bent inward. Lean forward gently from your hips towards your extended leg to stretch the hamstring. Hold, then switch legs.
- Cat-Camel Stretch (2 sets of 10 reps): Start in a tabletop position. Arch your back up, tucking your chin to your chest (Cat). Then, lower your stomach down, lifting your head and tailbone up (Camel). This helps increase spinal mobility.
- Chest Opener (2 sets of 30 seconds): Stand or sit upright. Clasp your hands behind your back and gently lift them, opening your chest. This stretch is excellent for improving upper body mobility and counteracting poor posture.
- Ankle Circles (2 sets of 10 reps each ankle): Sit or lie down and extend one leg. Rotate your ankle slowly in a circular motion. Switch directions after 5 reps. Repeat with the other ankle. This improves ankle mobility and reduces the risk of falls.

Cool-Down

- Walk for 5 minutes

30-60 seconds each:

- Standing Quadriceps Stretch
- Seated Hamstring Stretch

- Doorway Chest Stretch
- Seated Piriformis Stretch

Workout C: Lower Body Strength and Endurance

- Goblet Squats (3 sets of 8 -10 reps): Stand with your feet hip-width apart, holding a weight in front of your chest. Lower your body into a squat, keeping your chest lifted. Push back up to the starting position. This exercise targets your quadriceps, glutes, and hamstrings.
- Walking Lunges with Weights (3 sets of 10 reps each leg): Stand tall, holding a weight in each hand. Step forward with your right foot, lowering your body into a lunge. Push off your right foot to stand up, then repeat with the left foot. This exercise strengthens your lower body and challenges your balance and coordination.
- Calf Raises with Weights (3 sets of 15 reps): Stand holding a weight in each hand. Lift your heels off the ground, then lower them back down. This exercise strengthens your calf muscles.
- Single Leg Bridge (3 sets of 10 reps): Start lying on your back with your knees bent and feet flat on the ground. Next, lift one leg in the air so both thighs are level. Lift your hips up in the air through the leg on the ground while keeping your other leg extended straight in the air. Complete all reps, then repeat on the other side. This exercise targets your glutes, quads, core, and lower back.
- Wall Sit (2 sets of 30-60 seconds): Start with your back against a wall. Move your feet slightly forward. Slowly squat down to a challenging but doable position and maintain it for the duration of the exercise. Your back should remain against the wall throughout the exercise. This exercise targets your quadriceps.

Cool-Down:

- Walk for 5 minutes

30-60 seconds each:

- Standing Quadriceps Stretch
- Seated Hamstring Stretch
- Calf Stretch off step/stairs
- Doorway Chest Stretch

Workout D: Upper Body Strength and Endurance

Warm-Up (5 minutes): Start with a fast-paced walk, bike, or elliptical, then perform arm circles.

- Push-ups (2-3 sets of 10 reps). Perform on floor, bench, or wall.
- 1-Arm Dumbbell Back Rows (2-3 sets of 8-10 reps). Start by holding a dumbbell in one hand. Bend over at your hips while maintaining a flat back. For added support, place your other hand on a bench or chair. Row the dumbbell up to the side of your torso, then control back down. This exercise targets your back muscles.
- Half-Kneeling 1-Arm Shoulder Press (2-3 sets of 8-10 reps). Start in a half-kneeling position on the floor, with one knee on the ground while your other leg is up, your knee bent at 90 degrees, and your foot flat on the ground. Hold a dumbbell in your hand on the same side that your knee is on the ground. Perform a shoulder press. This exercise targets your shoulders, core, and hip stability.
- Dumbbell Bicep Curls (2-3 sets of 8-10 reps). While standing, hold dumbbells by your side. Bend your elbows up, then control back down. This exercise targets your biceps and forearms.
- Lying Dumbbell Tricep Extensions (2-3 sets of 8-10 reps). Start lying on your back. Grab a pair of dumbbells, then hold straight

up with your arms extended. Slowly bend your elbows and bring the dumbbells to the side of your head by your ears. Gently tap the floor, then extend your elbows back up. This exercise targets your triceps. Make sure to don't smash your face!

- 1-Arm Overhead Carry (3 sets of 30 seconds on each side). Start standing, holding a heavy dumbbell in the air with your arm straight. Then, walk for the duration of the exercise. Switch sides. Focus on maintaining an upright posture. This exercise targets your grip, core, shoulder stability, and balance.

Cool-Down:

- Walk for 5 minutes

30-60 seconds each:

- Doorway Chest Stretch
- Doorway Lat Stretch
- Wrist/Forearm flexor and extensor stretches

Remember to focus on performing each exercise with control and proper form. Rest for about one minute between sets to allow your muscles to recover. After each workout, cool down with walking, then some gentle stretching to promote flexibility and reduce muscle stiffness.

Don't forget to utilize your free copy of **5 Essential Daily Exercises for Posture** provided at the beginning of the book! Your cool-down is a perfect time to perform these exercises, as your body is warm and primed to increase mobility.

This advanced routine is designed to challenge you, push your boundaries, and take your strength training to the next level. Remember, it's not about perfection but progress. So, celebrate each workout, each lift, each rep. You're not just building muscles. You're building resilience, confidence, and a healthier, stronger you.

As we conclude this chapter, remember that strength training is a journey, not a destination. It's about embracing the process, celebrating progress, and continuously challenging yourself. So keep climbing, keep pushing, and keep believing in yourself. Your strength training peak is within reach, and the view from the top is absolutely worth it.

FREE ACCESS TO YOUR 4-WEEK STRENGTH TRAINING PROGRAM

Optimized for Seniors at Every Level - Beginner, Intermediate, and Advanced

Welcome to Your Journey to Strength and Vitality!

Are you ready to embark on a transformative journey that enhances your strength, balance, and overall well-being? Look no further! I'm excited to offer you free app access to your 4-Week Strength Training Program, exclusively designed for seniors.

Whether you're just starting out, have some experience, or are a seasoned exerciser, we have a program that fits your needs. Each program is crafted to help seniors like you optimize results, provide guidance every step of the way, and track progress over time.

What You'll Get:

- Flexible Workouts: Choose from the beginner, intermediate, or advanced programs provided in this book to match your fitness level.

- Easy-to-Follow Routines: Clear instructions and illustrations/videos help ensure you perform each exercise safely and effectively.
- Progress Tracking: Monitor your improvements week by week to stay motivated and see how far you've come.
- Community Support: Join our community of like-minded individuals who are on a similar journey of gaining strength and improving wellness

Program Overviews:

- Beginner: Designed for those new to strength training, focusing on basic movements to build a solid foundation.
- Intermediate: For those with some strength training experience, introducing more challenging exercises and techniques.
- Advanced: Tailored for experienced individuals, featuring intensive workouts for maximal strength and endurance gains.

How to Sign Up:

Simply scan the appropriate QR code below corresponding to the program level that suits you best. You'll receive immediate access to your 4-week strength training program. Create your account and get started today!

Click here for the beginner program!

Click here for the intermediate program!

Click here for the advanced program!

This is more than just a workout program; it's an opportunity to enhance your quality of life, boost your independence, and join a community that cheers you on. Embrace the chance to live your best life with strength and confidence. Sign up now and take the first step towards a stronger, healthier you!

KEEPING THE GAME ALIVE

Now that you've unlocked the secrets to improving strength and health in your senior years, it's time to share your newfound wisdom and guide others to this valuable resource.

By simply sharing your honest thoughts about this book on Amazon, you'll be pointing other seniors toward the guidance they need to embark on their own journey of strength training and healthier living.

Your opinion matters more than you might realize. It's not just a review; it's a beacon of hope for someone searching for a way to enhance their golden years. When you share your experience, you're not just recommending a book; you're endorsing a lifestyle change that could significantly improve someone's life.

Thank you for your invaluable contribution. We thrive when we pass on our knowledge and experiences – and your efforts are key in helping us achieve this.

Click here to leave your review on Amazon, or Scan the QR code below:

Every review counts, and yours could be the one that inspires another to take that first life-changing step toward a stronger, healthier future.

CONCLUSION

Conclusion

As we close the final pages of this book, let's take a moment to reflect on the journey we've embarked on together. We've explored the multifaceted world of strength training, demystified its myths, and celebrated its potential. We've learned that strength training, particularly for seniors, is not merely about lifting weights. It's about embracing a lifestyle that fosters health, vitality, and the joy of movement.

Your journey into strength training is a testament to your resilience, commitment, and desire to lead a healthy, vibrant life. Celebrate your progress, each rep, set, and workout completed. These are not just steps on your fitness journey but milestones on your path to improved health and longevity.

As you continue your strength training journey, remember that growth and progress come in many forms. It may be lifting a heavier weight, completing an additional rep, or simply feeling more energized and vibrant in your daily life. No matter how small, every step you take is a step towards a stronger, healthier you.

Your journey doesn't end here. This book has provided you with the foundational knowledge, strategies, and routines to kick-start your strength training journey. However, the world of strength training is vast and ever-evolving. I encourage you to continue learning, experimenting, and challenging yourself. Attend workshops, join fitness groups, and stay informed about the latest research in strength training.

Looking back on your journey, acknowledge your personal achievements. Whether it's sticking to your workout routine, mastering a new exercise, or noticing improvements in your strength and endurance. Each of these achievements is a testament to your effort, your dedication, and your ability to embrace new challenges.

Strength training for seniors is not just about building muscles. It's about building a lifestyle that fosters health, independence, and longevity. It's about embracing the joy of movement, the thrill of progress, and the power of resilience. As you continue your strength training journey, remember to celebrate each milestone, each victory, and each moment of growth.

Drawing inspiration from the words of Winston Churchill, "Success is not final, failure is not fatal: It is the courage to continue that counts." This powerful sentiment echoes through our exploration of strength training for seniors. As you step forward from this book, remember that your strength training journey is marked not just by successes but also by the challenges you face and overcome. Each session, each lift, and each moment of exertion is a testament to your courage and resilience. As you continue your journey, let this courage be your guide, propelling you toward a healthier, stronger, and more empowered self. Strength training is more than a physical activity; it's a courageous act of self-care and self-improvement."

Now, go gain confidence, vitality, and the power to live your best life. So here's to your strength, resilience, and unwavering spirit. Here's to your strength training journey and to the many victories and milestones that lie ahead. Keep lifting, keep growing, and keep shining. Your best life awaits.

REFERENCES

American Council on Exercise. (2016). Exercise Modifications and Variations. Retrieved from https://www.acefitness.org/education-and-resources/professional/ expert-articles/5903/exercise-modifications-and-variations/

American Council on Exercise. (2018). How Does Strength Training Increase Energy Levels? Retrieved from https://www.acefitness.org/education-and-resources/life style/blog/6468/how-does-strength-training-increase-energy-levels

American Heart Association. (2024, January 22). Celebrating Your Fitness Success. Retrieved from https://www.heart.org/en/healthy-living/fitness/staying-moti vated/celebrating-your-fitness-success

Arazi, H., Babaei, P., Moghimi, M., et al. (2021). Acute effects of strength and endurance exercise on serum BDNF and IGF-1 levels in older men. BMC Geriatrics, 21, 50. https://doi.org/10.1186/s12877-020-01937-6

Bedosky, L. (2018, October 18). 8 Best Fitness Apps for Older Adults. SilverSneakers. Retrieved from https://www.silversneakers.com/blog/8-best-fitness-apps-for-older-adults/

Bedosky, L. (2023, April 5). Strength Training for Older Adults: The SilverSneakers Guide. SilverSneakers. Retrieved from https://www.silversneakers.com/blog/why-older-adults-should-pick-up-strength-training/

Bubnis, D. (2023, March 27). Exercise Plan for Seniors: Strength, Stretching, and Balance. Healthline. Retrieved from https://www.healthline.com/health/every day-fitness/senior-workouts

Cannataro R, Cione E, Bonilla DA, Cerullo G, Angelini F, D'Antona G. (2022, July 18). Strength training in elderly: An useful tool against sarcopenia. Retrieved fromhttps://www.ncbi.nlm.nih.gov/pmc/articles/PMC9339797/

Centers for Disease Control and Prevention. Growing Stronger - Strength Training for Older Adults. Retrieved from https://www.cdc.gov/physicalactivity/down loads/growing_stronger.pdf

Consumer Reports. (2019, November 28). A Guide to Fitness Trackers for Seniors. Consumer Reports. Retrieved from https://www.consumerreports.org/electron ics-computers/fitness-trackers/fitness-trackers-for-seniors-a5305004198/

Corrigall, C. (2019, August 15). Overcoming Barriers to Elderly Exercise. Aegis Living. Retrieved from https://www.aegisliving.com/resource-center/overcoming-barri ers-to-exercise-among-the-elderly/

Deutz NE, Bauer JM, Barazzoni R, Biolo G, Boirie Y, Bosy-Westphal A, Cederholm T, Cruz-Jentoft A, Krznariç Z, Nair KS, Singer P, Teta D, Tipton K, Calder PC. (2014, April 24). Protein intake and exercise for optimal muscle function with aging: Recommendations from the ESPEN Expert Group. Retrieved fromhttps://www. ncbi.nlm.nih.gov/pmc/articles/PMC4208946/

Empowering the Elderly: Success Stories from Senior Fitness Training. American Sport and Fitness. Retrieved from https://www.americansportandfitness.com/blogs/fitness-blog/empowering-the-elderly-success-stories-from-senior-fitness-training

Fien S, Linton C, Mitchell JS, Wadsworth DP, Szabo H, Askew CD, Schaumberg MA. (2022, February 12). Characteristics of community-based exercise programs for older adults with chronic diseases: A systematic scoping review. Aging Clin Exp Res. 34(7): 1511–1528. Retrieved from https://www.ncbi.nlm.nih.gov/pmc/articles/PMC8852913/

Fiatarone, M. A., O'Neill, E. F., Ryan, N. D., Clements, K. M., Solares, G. R., Nelson, M. E., ... & Evans, W. J. (1994). Exercise training and nutritional supplementation for physical frailty in very elderly people. New England Journal of Medicine, 330(25), 1769-1775.

Fetters, K. (2013, May 19). 5 Strength Training Exercises for Seniors: Everything You Need to Know. SilverSneakers. Retrieved from https://www.silversneakers.com/blog/strength-training-for-seniors/

Fragala, M; Cadore, E; Dorgo, S; Izquierdo, M; Kraemer, W; Peterson, M; Ryan, P. (2019). Resistance Training for Older Adults: Position Statement. The Journal of Strength and Conditioning Research. Retrieved from https://www.nsca.com/contentassets/2a4112fb355a4a48853bbafbe070fb8e/resistance_training_for_older_adults__position.1.pdf

Freytag C. (2022, February 4). 20-Minute Strength Training Workout for Seniors. Very well Fit. Retrieved from https://www.verywellfit.com/20-minute-senior-weight-training-workout-3498676

Garone, S. (2021, September 30). How to Adapt Your Fitness Routine as You Age. Healthline. Retrieved from https://www.healthline.com/health/the-definitive-guide-to-adapting-your-fitness-routine-for-every-phase-of-life

Häkkinen, K., Pakarinen, A., Hannonen, P., Häkkinen, A., Airaksinen, O., Valkeinen, H., & Alen, M. (2002). Effects of strength training on muscle strength, cross-sectional area, maximal electromyographic activity, and serum hormones in premenopausal women with fibromyalgia. The Journal of Rheumatology, 29(6), 1287-1295.

Harvard Health Publishing. (2018). How strength training helps you live longer. Retrieved from https://www.health.harvard.edu/staying-healthy/how-strength-training-helps-you-live-longer

Harvard Health Publishing. (2018). Weight lifting can boost your mental health. Retrieved from https://www.health.harvard.edu/mind-and-mood/weight-lifting-can-boost-your-mental-health

Harvard Health Publishing. (2022, January 16). Strength training builds more than muscles. Retrieved from https://www.health.harvard.edu/staying-healthy/strength-training-builds-more-than-muscles

Harvard Health Publishing. (2022, March 14). The importance of stretching. Retrieved from https://www.health.harvard.edu/staying-healthy/the-importance-of-stretching

Hart PD, Buck DJ. (2019, January 23). The effect of resistance training on health-related quality of life in older adults: a systematic review. Health Promot Perspect. Retrieved from https://www.ncbi.nlm.nih.gov/pmc/articles/PMC6377696/

Hart, PD; Buck, DJ.. (2019, January 23). The effect of resistance training on health-related quality of life in older adults. Health Promot Perspect. Retrieved from https://www.ncbi.nlm.nih.gov/pmc/articles/PMC6377696/

Harvard T.H. Chan School of Public Health. (2022, August 2024). Positive attitude about aging could boost health. Retrieved from https://www.hsph.harvard.edu/news/hsph-in-the-news/positive-attitude-about-aging-could-boost-health/

Hayes EJ, Stevenson E, Sayer AA, Granic A, Hurst C. (2023). Recovery from Resistance Exercise in Older Adults. A Systematic Scoping Review. Sports Med Open. Retrieved from https://www.ncbi.nlm.nih.gov/pmc/articles/PMC10317890/

How Technology Can Help To Improve Strength Training. ShapeScale. Retrieved from https://shapescale.com/blog/20-minute-fitness-podcast/technology-to-improve-your-strength-training/

How to Set SMART Goals for Strength Training. Barbell Logic. Retrieved from https://barbell-logic.com/smart-goals-for-strength/

Jackson, E. A., et al. (2020). Nurturing Career Development for Human Sustainable Development. Retrieved fromhttps://core.ac.uk/download/483650110.pdf

Johns Hopkins Medicine. Fall Prevention: Balance and Strength Exercises for Older Adults. Retrieved from https://www.hopkinsmedicine.org/health/wellness-and-prevention/fall-prevention-exercises

Judge LW, Bellar DM, Popp JK, Craig BW, Schoeff MA, Hoover DL, Fox B, Kistler BM, Al-Nawaiseh AM. (2021, July 28). Hydration to Maximize Performance and Recovery: Knowledge, Attitudes, and Behaviors Among Collegiate Track and Field Throwers. Journal of Human Kinetics. Retrieved from https://www.ncbi.nlm.nih.gov/pmc/articles/PMC8336541/

Latham, N. K., Anderson, C. S., Lee, A., Bennett, D. A., Moseley, A., & Cameron, I. D. (2003). A randomized, controlled trial of quadriceps resistance exercise and vitamin D in frail older people: The Frailty Interventions Trial in Elderly Subjects (FITNESS). Journal of the American Geriatrics Society, 51(3), 291-299.

Liu-Ambrose, T., Nagamatsu, L. S., Graf, P., Beattie, B. L., Ashe, M. C., & Handy, T. C. (2010). Resistance training and executive functions: A 12-month randomized controlled trial. Archives of Internal Medicine, 170(2), 170-178.

Mayer F, Scharhag-Rosenberger F, Carlsohn A, Cassel M, Müller S, Scharhag J.. (2011, May 27). The Intensity and Effects of Strength Training in the Elderly. Dtsch Arztebl Int. Retrieved from https://www.ncbi.nlm.nih.gov/pmc/articles/PMC3117172/

Mayo Clinic. (2021). Exercise: 7 benefits of regular physical activity. Retrieved from https://www.mayoclinic.org/healthy-lifestyle/fitness/in-depth/exercise/art-20048389

Mayo Clinic. (2022, November 29). Weight training: Do's and don'ts of proper technique. Retrieved from https://www.mayoclinic.org/healthy-lifestyle/fitness/in-depth/weight-training/art-20045842

Mayo Clinic. Aerobic exercise: How to warm up and cool down. Retrieved from https://www.mayoclinic.org/healthy-lifestyle/fitness/in-depth/exercise/art-20045517

McManus, M. (2023, July 21). What's more important as you age — stretching, balance... CNN. Retrieved from https://www.cnn.com/2023/07/21/health/exercises-for-aging-bodies-wellness/index.html

MD Anderson Cancer Center. (2016, May). The truth behind six strength training myths. Retrieved from https://www.mdanderson.org/publications/focused-on-health/thetruthbehindsixstrengthtrainingmyths.h12-1590624.html

National Council on Aging. (2022). Falls Prevention Facts. Retrieved from https://www.ncoa.org/article/falls-prevention-facts

National Institute on Aging. (2021, January 2). Vitamins and Minerals for Older Adults. Retrieved from https://www.nia.nih.gov/health/vitamins-and-supplements/vitamins-and-minerals-older-adults

National Institute on Aging. (2021, November 23). Healthy Meal Planning: Tips for Older Adults. Retrieved from https://www.nia.nih.gov/health/healthy-eating-nutrition-and-diet/healthy-meal-planning-tips-older-adults

National Institute on Aging. (2022, June 30). How can strength training build healthier bodies as we age? Retrieved from https://www.nia.nih.gov/news/how-can-strength-training-build-healthier-bodies-we-age

OpenAI. (2024). ChatGPT (4) [Large language model]. https://chat.openai.com

Peri, C. (2021, November 18). Relieve Aches and Pain, Aging, Home Tips. WebMD. Retrieved from https://www.webmd.com/pain-management/caregiver-pain-relief

Phillips, H. (2023, February 20). 12 Everyday Household Items That Double as Gym Equipment. CNET. Retrieved from https://www.cnet.com/health/fitness/12-everyday-household-items-for-your-workouts/

Portela, A. (2023, September 29). Home Gym Setup for Seniors: Creating a Safe and Effective Space. GinaST.com. Retrieved from https://ginast.com/home-gym-setup-for-seniors/

Rischer, B. (2018, February 7). The 7-Minute Yoga Flow for Older Adults. SilverSneakers. Retrieved from https://www.silversneakers.com/blog/yoga-seniors-7-minute-flow-ease-stress-increase-flexibility/

Robinson L, Smith M, Segal J. (2024, January 5). Senior Exercise and Fitness Tips. HelpGuide. Retrieved from https://www.helpguide.org/articles/healthy-living/exercise-and-fitness-as-you-age.htm

Schuler, L. (2017, August 30). Preventing Strength Training Injuries for Older Adults. SilverSneakers. Retrieved from https://www.silversneakers.com/blog/prevent-strength-training-injuries/

Senior Helpers. (2023, September 19). Leading by Example: Fitness Routines for Caregivers. Senior Helpers. Retrieved from https://www.seniorhelpers.com/ca/pleasanton/resources/blogs/2023-09-19/

Seguin R, Epping J, Buchner D, Bloch R, Nelson M. Centers for Disease Control and Prevention. Growing Stronger - Strength Training for Older Adults. Retrieved from https://www.cdc.gov/physicalactivity/downloads/growing_stronger.pdf

Shadbolt, J. (2019, November 6). 8 Low-Impact Workouts and Exercises for Seniors. SilverSneakers. Retrieved from https://www.silversneakers.com/blog/low-impact-workouts-older-adults/

Sherrington, C., Fairhall, N. J., Wallbank, G. K., Tiedemann, A., Michaleff, Z. A., Howard, K., ... & Lord, S. R. (2019). Exercise for preventing falls in older people living in the community. Cochrane Database of Systematic Reviews, (1).

Singh, N. A., Clements, K. M., & Fiatarone, M. A. (1997). A randomized controlled trial of the effect of exercise on sleep. Sleep, 20(2), 95-101.

Stathokostas L, Little RM, Vandervoort AA, Paterson DH. (2012, November 8). Flexibility Training and Functional Ability in Older Adults.J Aging Res. Retrieved from https://www.ncbi.nlm.nih.gov/pmc/articles/PMC3503322/

Team Trainerize. (2023, July 20). 9 of the Best Remote Personal Trainer Platforms. Trainerize. Retrieved from https://www.trainerize.com/blog/remote-personal-trainer-platforms/

The Art of Manliness. (2016, February 3). The Ultimate Glossary of Strength and Conditioning Terms. Retrieved from https://www.artofmanliness.com/health-fitness/fitness/the-ultimate-glossary-of-strength-and-conditioning-terms/

Verimatrix Cybersecurity. (2021, January 29). How to Keep Fitness App Data Safe and Secure. Verimatrix. Retrieved from https://www.verimatrix.com/cybersecurity/knowledge-base/how-to-protect-sensitive-user-data-with-fitness-app-security/

WebMD. (2022, November 29). Best Balance Exercises for Seniors. WebMD. Retrieved from https://www.webmd.com/healthy-aging/best-balance-exercises-for-seniors

Westcott, W. L. (2012). Resistance training is medicine: Effects of strength training on health. Current Sports Medicine Reports, 11(4), 209-216.